Praise for
SHE'LL BE HOME IN THE SPRINGTIME

"*She'll Be Home in the Springtime* is both insightful and easy to read. Special education has come a long way, yet not far enough. We are better at delivering services to the more "typical" diagnoses, yet still struggling to find the "right" methods and services for those who don't quite fit into the box. The author was leading the way in delivering and receiving and advocating so strongly for Cait. I loved reading all the details, the struggles and joys in Cait's accomplishments!"

Grace Jang
Senior Curriculum Coordinator, Birch Family Services

"As a school psychologist, I'm privy to the concerns of parents as they internalize the life-changing information that comes with their child's Asperger's Syndrome diagnosis. *She'll Be Home in the Springtime* gives an authentic longitudinal accounting, written by the mother of a daughter with Asperger's, in a inviting yet no-holds bar manner. Ms. Ujlaky shares what she refers to as her journey; from her first sensing that something in Cait "was not right" through the pitfalls of varied diagnoses, and ultimately preparing her child for an independent life. The author captures what it's like to be a forerunner in the years that preceded school awareness of Asperger's, as well as educational reluctance to comply with new standard practices. This is not a diatribe, but rather a hosanna to the intrepid family and friends whose convictions never swayed. I heartily recommend *She'll Be Home in the Springtime* for families and support team members of all special needs children."

David S. Leslie-Skaller
M.S.E, NASP, New York City Dep't of Education

"In addition to assisting parents and teachers, *She'll Be Home in the Springtime* benefits health professionals as well. It gives readers insider perspectives on what it's like to raise children with spectrum disorders as well as other disabilities. This book fills a much-needed void and is valuable to anyone working with children who are not typical."

Ellen Heudeska
R.N. Pediatrics

"*She'll Be Home in the Springtime* takes the reader, whether that is a parent, teacher, sibling, or stranger, on a beautiful and metaphoric, yet real journey, from the perspective of a family and an individual living with an autism spectrum disorder. This journey spans moments of beautiful celebrations, wit's end, and incredible frustrations—all a part of honoring Cait's perspective and life."

Laura Bonazinga Bouyea
M.S., SLP-CCC Autism Consultant, Social Coach

"The author's journey with her daughter is expressed in a very entertaining voice—painted in vivid vignettes and generous sprinkles of humor. From Lyn Ujlaky's story, other parents will derive advice, comfort, and a license to laugh at themselves, while enjoying their own children's talents and foibles. At the same time they will find themselves exerting the amazing energy it takes to be, as the author describes it, 'Knights of the Roundtable.' "

Glenna Giveans
Learning Specialist, Davis Autism/ADHD Facilitator

She'll Be Home in the Springtime

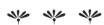

The Story of a Mother, a Daughter, and Asperger's

Lyn Elizabeth Ujlaky

published by

Flynn and Park Street Press
144 Hominy Pot Road
Post Office Box 1781
New London, New Hampshire 03257
www.flynnandparkstreetpress.com

Book design: Linda Tyler
Cover photograph : Cuttyhunk Island, MA, 1994

NOTE TO THE READER
This book is a memoir. The individuals, conversations, and locations portrayed
here are how I remember them. In order to maintain anonymity, I've changed
the names of people and places along with many identifying characteristics and
details. So while much of the retelling is based in fact, the privacy of individuals and the institutions involved have been protected to the best of my ability.

PUBLISHER'S CATALOGING-IN-PUBLICATION

Ujlaky, Lyn Elizabeth
  She'll be home in the springtime : the story of a mother, a daughter, and
Asperger's / Lyn Elizabeth Ujlaky

LCCN 2014909015
ISBN 978-0-9903233-5-8
ISBN 978-0-9903233-6-5
1. Ujlaky, Lyn Elizabeth. 2. Parenting—Asperger's—Memoir 3. Education
    I. Title

                                                                    616.85

ISBN 978-0-9903233-5-8

Dedicated to my daughters:

Courtney - who was the first to hold her sister,
and has championed her ever since.

Cait - who taught us all to listen,
and then to listen again.

Acknowledgements

While I journeyed through uncharted, and sometimes-rough waters, while raising my daughter, Cait, I had an army of real, live angels who traveled with me. During those early intervention years, when my story with Cait began to unfold, her daycare providers and the early childhood specialists were there, guiding me. They provided Cait with a foundation for all her future learning experiences. Our medical community remained unfailing in their professional and thoughtful approach while treating Cait and monitoring her progress over many years. Each time one moved away, I mourned their loss as though they were family. Special gratitude goes to Drs. Diane Kittredge and Paolo Bentivoglio, whom we'd have followed to the ends of the earth if we could.

Cait's teachers, throughout elementary and high school, were her champions. An arduous student, she'd constantly provide them with new learning curves, but at no time did any of them give up. They were always available, helping and challenging Cait to do her best.

I'm not sure I would have been able to remain on our trajectory if it weren't for psychologist, Janine Scheiner, whose humor and talent were the glue that held us together. I'll always be thankful to her speech and language pathologists. Katie Willard's approaches led us to Michelle Garcia Winner and her innovative Social Thinking program, where Cait learned perspective taking in creative and meaningful ways. Klaren Warner reentered Cait's life, after first meeting her at age three, and pulled together a group of students and parents that met socially after school for years, giving this unique group of teens a chance to practice their skills in a friendly environment. Years later, this group of now young adults and their parents still connect through the generous spirit of Candie Darcy and son, Nathan.

Cait, also, had many devoted educational assistants over the years. They never stopped believing in Cait and unfailingly worked on her behalf.

Her Crafty Girls' leader and close friend, Patty Charyk, impacted Cait in profound ways that still echo today.

This book would never have been written without the encouragement and support of a wide group of colleagues and close friends. The Ray Writers group started this book. They informed me over coffee at Bumplebys that my stab at an article on Asperger's was actually my own story waiting to be written. It was at the Writer's Center in White River Junction, Vermont, under Joni Cole's tutorage, and the feedback of its participants, where I began to take their suggestion of turning my work into an account of parenting a child with Asperger's seriously. Author Katharine Britton and her memoir group, Sonja Swierczynski and Judy Miller, helped me flush it out. Finally, my dearest friend and soul sister, Adrienne, pushed me to complete it. An author herself, she'd read each chapter, help me tear it apart again and again, and then offered ways to put it back together so that anyone reading would travel each path alongside me.

As this book got closer to completion, I pulled together 'my magnificent seven'—Hatsy McGraw, Deb Franzoni, Ginger Wallis, Patty Charyk, Jan Scheiner, Katie Willard, and Alice Eberhardt - writers, professionals, friends, and fact checkers, who took the time to proof and offer up their suggestions. Gina Ottoboni, an amazing copy editor, took my book to the next level through her editorial talents and attention to detail.

But in truth, it was my family who really wrote this story. Our combined memories filled its pages with humor and love. My mom taught me that angels really do exit as she continues to watch over Cait and me. When I'm at my wits end, I can hear her words of wisdom and feel her anchor me, yet again. My dad, at ninety-one, unfailingly continues to support and applaud his youngest grandchild. Cait's stepdad, Mike, is the one among us who truly gets Cait, and remains loyal to everything quirky and different about her. He's the first to get her jokes, and can remember the same funny line from a movie they've seen together years before. Stepsister, Sam, was Cait's first friend, and though they travel separate paths now, Sam makes sure their lives still cross when they're able. Courtney remains the world's most remarkable sister. She's the ultimate confidant every girl wants and what I dreamt a sister could be.

And then there's Cait—unforgettable and irreplaceable. If I was meant to take this journey, I couldn't have picked a better companion.

Contents

PART III – Dance Upon the Mountains

PROLOGUE

When Cait was born, I understood pure bliss. I had wanted a second baby even before I gave birth to my first. Growing up an only child, I craved a sibling, the one person whose bond couldn't be broken. I had missed sharing secrets and having a built-in companion, so I refused to consider that my own daughter might experience a similar fate. My family, of course, was full of their own advice.

"You should be grateful, you already have a beautiful daughter." My mother's words were meant to comfort. They didn't.

My religious and childless aunt tried to guide me, "It's in God's hands. If you were meant to have more children, you would." I smiled politely and nodded.

I didn't think of myself as greedy, and why would God frown on me for wanting a second baby? When my body failed to deliver, my husband and I decided to adopt. Our Vermont adoption agency connected us with a birth mother.

Cait was born the beginning of May, but state law required a two-week wait period. Mother's Day fell within that time frame, and I was convinced the sentimental holiday would change the birth mother's mind. But after fourteen days of labor pains, our family was driving north to Burlington, Vermont, to meet our new daughter and sister.

It couldn't have been a more beautiful spring day. Courtney, almost seven, sat in the backseat clutching a newborn outfit she had specially picked out. We were ahead of schedule, yet as eager as I was to finally meet my new daughter, I didn't mind waiting a little longer. I loved the feeling of anticipation, the sensation that something wonderful was about to happen. We decided to stop at the University of Vermont's campus, my husband's alma mater. Browsing the bookstore we found a UVM infant T-shirt and bought it on the spot. Then we drove to fetch the little girl who would change our lives forever.

Like all moms, I thought my new baby was exquisite. Her eyes, wide and a deep blue-gray, complimented her small features and the blonde wisps that framed her face. She had an agreeable disposition from the start. Cait rarely cried. Before long, she was even sleeping through the night.

Courtney, the first to hold her, immediately fell in love with her new, real live doll. That first week Cait was her sister's show-and-tell at school, and by week two she was mine. I was working as a resource-room teacher for a school district that didn't provide adoption leave. At the end of the school year, I had meetings and reports, so as I typed, I balanced Cait on my lap. My room was decked out with a small travel playpen and rocking chair. Cait unofficially became the school's mascot.

Like clockwork, each day at 11:30 a colleague on lunch detail would appear, gently lift Cait with one arm while grabbing her bright yellow infant seat in the other. "We're off!" she'd call, before I had a chance to protest. Cait was now part of her lunch shift.

One morning during the second-grade Colonial Days Festival, I dropped Cait off at a nearby homestead—a 1776 reproduction of a settler's cabin built close to the school grounds. The teacher placed her in a wooden cradle to the delight of the children as they cross-stitched and made cornhusk dolls. Separation was never an issue. I left her there, smugly accepting that my Cait could be passed from person to person, never fussing or complaining, but accepting each new pair of hands that held her. Even the school's most challenging boy liked nothing better than to stop by and rock her every afternoon. His reward was the contentment on her face. Cait seemed to know what he needed. Later on, I'd attribute Cait's rare absences from school to her first six weeks of life when she was exposed to every elementary school microbe. They made her own immune system hum.

The early morning hours, late that spring, were my alone time with her. We'd often just sit and rock listening to the birds' first song of the day. I'd reflect on how many heartstrings she tugged since her arrival. Cait's sweet nature made her easy to love. I felt blessed. As I contemplated her future, I rarely considered my own. I wouldn't realize until years later how my life as a parent would take me on a journey I was neither expecting, nor prepared for. Maybe *pure bliss* was in not knowing what lay ahead.

Part I

INTO THE FRAY

"Once more into the fray.
  Into the last good fight I'll ever know ..."

From the movie, *The Grey*, by director Joe Carnahan

.

1

CONNECTING THE DOTS

Trot trot to Boston
Trot trot to Lynn
Watch out baby Cait
Or you'll fall in

It was time for Cait's well child visit. Left in Dr. Erickson's exam room, I bounced Cait, now two, on the edge of my knees chanting her favorite song. When I got to the last word, "in," I let her drop down through my legs just inches from the floor. She'd squeal and beg for more. I kept the rhythm going, never taking my eyes off the door. If Erickson didn't appear soon, I'd be his patient instead of my toddler. I was tired of the game, but knew stopping wasn't an option or she'd squirm off my lap and take off. Now that Cait was mobile, anything within her reach was fair game. I could calm her with a picture book. I scanned the room—nothing. He calls himself a pediatrician? A hundred versions of the "Trot, Trot" song beat running in circles, but it was taking its toll. Still, I continued the chant, each time dropping her faster, ready to scream, "What the hell is taking so long?"

The doctor must have heard my silent plea. The door opened. He sat down opposite us and smiled, "And how's Cait today?" He extended his stethoscope for her to hold before he listened to her heart. I wanted to snatch it and put it up to my own, now racing.

As he leaned into Cait, she giggled and nestled further into my lap.

"Dr. Erickson, something's not right."

"What? Terrible twos getting to you?" He smiled, entered some numbers on Cait's chart and pulled the scope out of his ears.

"Tell me about it." I knew the man who filled the doorframe and looked like a Norwegian Viking saw a healthy, spunky two-year old.

"She's like a motor that doesn't stop." Was he getting this? "She puts everything in her mouth, even the sand at the beach." Now he'll understand. "She doesn't ask for a cookie or even point, but she climbs her way to the top of a cabinet and takes one." I ended just as my breath ran out.

"Active doesn't mean something's wrong. A child with any type of attention problems wouldn't be able to sit in your lap for more than five minutes."

I glanced down at the top of her head as she sucked on the pacifier I still couldn't get her to give up.

I felt foolish. "She's so rambunctious. She hardly talks."

"Cait looks fine. Continue to keep an eye on things. We'll chat again at her next visit." He indulged me like I was a hypochondriac.

Walking out I managed the door with Cait held tightly in my arms. I nestled my nose against her cheek and drank in her soft, still-baby scent. "Mommy loves you, Caity. Mommy loves you a lot." With that she tightened her small arms around me, too.

Not long after our visit to Dr. Erickson, Cait's day care provider pulled me aside. Mother of four, Hannah was a no-nonsense, spirited woman. I was over the moon the day I snatched up her services shortly after Cait's arrival into our lives. She lived in a large, welcoming, old, white colonial. The beautiful, well-planned gardens that bordered her walkways were in full bloom from early spring until the first frost. I felt like I had found a tailored-down version of the Waltons. A special education teacher by training, Hannah decided to be at home with her children and took in a few more for extra income. I loved the energy she gave to everything around her.

When Cait started at Hannah's, at the age of six months, Hannah was taking care of two children just a few months older than Cait. My daughter was now part of a bustling household brimming with activity and opportunities for reciprocal play, but Cait didn't seem to absorb any of it. Compared to Hannah's own children and the two toddlers in her care, Cait's differences became pronounced.

After school one day, Hannah had me sit in the garden with her as we watched Cait and the others playing. She echoed the concerns I had shared with Dr. Erickson months earlier. "Maybe it's nothing, but I'm seeing her get more frustrated each time she wants something someone else has."

I felt a lump in my throat. I had seen it too. She put her hand over mine.

I was strangely relieved that someone else was finally echoing the concerns I had attempted to share that day in Dr. Erickson's office. Yet hearing them left me worried. I was sad to think that the little girl dressed in Osh Kosh overalls, and digging in the sand, would somehow miss out on reaching all the childhood milestones like everyone else.

On Hannah's suggestion, I started looking for a formal preschool that might benefit Cait. Staying home was never an option. We needed two salaries. I placed her name on the wait list of a reputable daycare center that took children from infancy through age five. I was grateful when a few months later a spot opened for three days a week. On the other two she continued at Hannah's.

It didn't take long before her preschool teachers were asking the same questions.

Cait was a revved up engine. She would hardly look in your direction if you spoke to her and she'd answer a question with a question. The frustration Hannah noticed was turning into aggression.

Trish, the director, called me in. I liked her and I knew she cared about Cait. She didn't hold anything back, starting with the center's ritual morning circle. "Cait rolls around and refuses to sit up and participate. It's disruptive to everyone."

It appeared that mornings went quickly downhill from there. If someone wanted a toy and Cait wasn't ready to give it up, she settled it with a clunk over her classmate's head. Any type of art activity always dissolved into tears. When the staff tried to calm her, they felt like they were speaking to her in foreign tongues. She relaxed during naptime only if they let her fall asleep with a book.

"What would you like me to do?" I was at a loss.

In a blink, Trish was helping to navigate us into the local Early Essential Ed program designed to catch early developmental concerns. While Cait was tested and observed, they provided support and suggestions to her providers. Around the same time, I changed pediatricians. I liked Dr. Erickson, but he and I were on a different page. I didn't have the time for him to catch up.

Cait had a jumpstart in a system meant to detect and address all my early concerns and those of her teachers. She was eligible for services in the areas of language and motor skills. Claire, a speech and language pathologist, arrived at the day care and worked with Cait to build her vocabulary and help her begin to follow multi-step directions. Cait was now being taught how to take turns instead of hitting and screaming. Visual aids were used to assist her when transitioning from one activity to the next. An occupational therapist addressed her fine and gross motor skills. She had her stringing beads and she rolled on a scooter board with a beanbag on her back for balance and sensory feedback. My own vocabulary was about to grow as well. I learned that Cait craved proprioceptive input, or sensations from her muscles and joints, which in turn increased body awareness. Now Cait's delight in roughhousing with her sister's older friends made sense. She loved being tackled and squeezed when they played a mock game of football with her.

Like everyone else on Cait's new day care team, I was beginning to make sense of Cait's odd quirks. As a little girl, Cait could never leave the local K-Mart shopping plaza without insisting on riding the small carousel right outside the store. As soon she was up on her pony and the quarters were in the slot, she'd wrap her arms around its plastic mane and tuck her chin to one side, tight against her shoulder. The entire time the ponies circled around with the music playing, Cait didn't budge from this position. Someone else looking on would have thought the frightened-looking girl was having her first pony ride, not her hundredth. It was another sign of her challenges with sensory processing. Cait's vestibular system, responsible for her sense of balance, was under activated. So now when we visited the Occupational Therapist's office, she couldn't wait until she was strapped in the large trapeze-like swing and spun in circles. Cait was seeking out ways to focus herself. Cait's new regime consisted of a wide-array of sensory feedback activities from blowing on whistles to jumping on trampolines to hiking with weights in her pack.

One day while I was vacuuming Claire called. Cait picked up the phone. "Is your mom home?"

"No," Cait answered, "She'll be home in the springtime," and immediately hung up.

A day later when Claire reached me, we couldn't help but laugh, but deep inside it concerned me. It was another example of Cait's language deficits. It reminded me once again that there was still a lot of work ahead, but I finally had a team of professionals to help connect the dots. Just as I was beginning to let a sense of relief replace my worries, it all changed direction.

I was at a meeting with two of Cait's service providers and Trish.

"We're thinking that perhaps Cait is showing signs of pervasive developmental disorder," shared her occupational therapist.

It sounded terrible. I had a million questions, but not one would leave my mouth.

"Her delayed development and things, such as her lack of toilet training, could be indicators of something more serious," said Trish.

"What are you telling me?" Trying to keep the panic out of my voice, I was convinced they were giving me a death sentence. All dreams of normalcy were crumbling.

I immediately brought these latest concerns up with Cait's new pediatrician, Susan. "Lyn, I'm certain, Cait doesn't fall into this category. I'm sending you an article on the disorder. Tell me what you think."

After reading the piece, I came to understand that the term pervasive was used to describe a group of disorders—one of which was autism. I realized Cait's day care team was hesitant to use the word autistic, but I could sense they were worried that Cait's developmental delays might be an early sign for the most serious of the pervasive development disorders. I had gone from Dr. Erickson, who said nothing was wrong, to a team of professionals suggesting my three-year-old might be trapped for life in a world only known to her. I blessed Susan for her candidness and insight. I refused to connect that dot. In my heart, I knew this was not my Cait.

After that, I learned to listen to my own voice. A few months later Cait was toilet-trained. The school staff found that having Cait sit in her teacher's lap during circle time helped increase her sensory diet. Hugging her had a calming effect and kept her from becoming too antsy. A steno pad began traveling back and forth between preschool and home. If the staff could communicate details about her day, it might inspire conversation. There were times I got more information than I wanted and it kept me up at night. Yet, Cait's conversation skills improved. Her beloved *Triceratops* and *T. rex* plastic toys were now talking to each other.

Though Cait made gains, she still lagged behind her peers. New specialists were suggested in an effort to discover something that might have been overlooked. Their evaluations didn't provide anything new or conclusive.

Somewhere along the way I found myself sitting across from Dr. Cooper, a child development specialist. He confirmed Cait's challenges: understanding oral directions and integrating what she saw into a motor task, like copying a shape. Everything he noted, I already knew. But, he also surprised me by pointing out her energy and delightful imagination.

"Cait wanted to be in charge of all the interactions during our testing," he smiled, "It might have interfered with some of her performance on the tests." He shared that her meltdowns were probably Cait attempting to manage the information coming her way so it was less overwhelming and confusing.

As our conversation was nearing an end, he sheepishly smiled across the table at me. "You know, Cait was born two hundred years too late. In a different time and place, her active nature and take-charge spirit would have won her the West."

"So that's all I need to do," I smiled, "Just turn back the clock."

While Cait's behaviors were being documented and reports were being written, I found that my husband and I were drifting further apart. His job kept him working long hours away from home. He was becoming less and less available to our family. The decision to divorce came as no surprise to either of us. But the day I walked down the court steps, I was gripped with the sudden panic that I was now sole navigator in the lives of both my daughters. I reflected back on Dr. Cooper's comment that day about Cait winning the West. Maybe he was right. Cait was simply Cait. And even if I could connect some dots for my daughter, I couldn't connect them all.

2

THE GREAT CUPCAKE BATTLE

Hannigan's was my local grocery and safe haven—one of those small-town markets that is an anomaly in a world of super-sized grocery stores. For me it was the perfect quick stop with short lines. It's how I did most of my shopping when I had Cait in tow.

Large stores took too long, and she was a magnet for everything sugar-coated. I'd always end up at the register with several items I didn't remember putting in my cart. The bright lighting and volume of customers seemed to set off a primal trigger in Cait. She'd lean all the way back in the grocery cart's child seat, bracing her hands on the bar in front, until she was practically upside down in an effort to escape. And there was always something we'd pass that she had to have. I'd walk through the aisles continuously weighing my options. If I denied her, was the ensuing battle worth it? I'd seen other supermarket meltdowns with tear-streaked children being dragged beside pale, stricken parents. I was unashamedly embarrassed for them, and often annoyed by their lack of parenting skills. Yet, here I was with my own grocery-store nightmare. Pay back was a bitch.

Pulling into Hannigan's, I'd count the number of cars in the lot and then estimate the length of the line. I'd race through the narrow aisles on worn linoleum floors, and pick up only necessities. Sometimes I wasn't fast enough for Cait who'd eye some prize she couldn't leave without. There was rarely more than one register open, but I always felt the locals, who shopped this market for generations, had heard their share of disgruntled children. Waiting in this line I never felt like I stood out.

Once, I timed it all wrong. It was late in the day. We were both tired, but out of milk. It seemed like everyone else had the same idea. I was trapped in line with someone I didn't recognize running the register. She was having a conversation with each customer, and would stop and check prices from time to time. I felt everything go into slow motion. My impatience began to surface. I tried gently tapping my foot and taking deep breaths. Cait broke away from my hold only to return a second later with a cellophane bag that held two chocolate cupcakes. I scowled my disapproval. She smiled back and put them on the register's conveyor belt.

Cait's brilliance was in her willfulness, which trumped everything else. Her language skills might have lagged behind her peers, but she usually knew how to get her way. Sometimes, I thought she didn't use words to ask because she didn't want to hear, "No," for an answer. Once, when denied an action figure in a toy store she threw it and several others off the shelf in frustration. She looked like a Sci Fi robot with loose, frayed wires, popping and sizzling. Hers was a sensory system on constant overload. I knew her poor conversation skills left her frustrated. She lacked the power of persuasion.

She could never argue why a package of cupcakes had a rightful place in the cart along with everything else. Yet though she wasn't able to get out the right words at the right moment, she damn well knew when her mother was trapped in the checkout line. I looked at the snake of tired shoppers behind me, and let her package go through along with the milk, but at that moment we had declared war.

Outside Hannigan's I silently buckled her into her car seat in the back and placed the bag up front. I got into the driver's seat and slowly drove out of the lot. Instead of turning at our road, I drove straight ahead and turned a deaf ear to her demands for her prized treat. "Mommy's stopping at your sister's school first, Cait." My voice was calm and alien, almost sounding like I'd been sedated.

Her tears stopped.

"Cait, I never said it was okay to buy those cupcakes, did I?" Our eyes locked in the rear view mirror.

I turned into the deserted elementary school parking lot and drove to the end of the schoolyard where the large, green steel dumpster stood. I pulled up in front of it, got out of my car with the package of cupcakes, and tossed them in. Watching the cupcakes sink lower into a sea of colored construction paper and crumpled lunch wrappers rid me of all my pent up tension and anger. I got back in the car.

Cait arched her back against the child seat and let out a blood-curdling wail, "Give me them! Give me them!" she repeated at the top of her lungs.

I ignored her screams. "Don't ever do that again, Cait."

I'm not sure she heard me through her tantrum, but I felt a hell of a lot better. It didn't last long. Even though I had won this cup-cake battle, I knew I was losing the war.

3

MORE CASUALTIES

At the end of every fall season, our town held their annual ski sale. Courtney, Cait's older sister, was always right on it. A born athlete, there wasn't a season or a sport she didn't participate in. The ski sale was her opportunity to make sure she had all the equipment she'd need for the upcoming winter. It started at noon, and to help offset the expense, we'd bring in our own outgrown skis and skates to sell earlier in the day. The logical side of me knew it would be challenging for three-and-a-half-year-old Cait, but this was important to her sister. As both hands struck twelve, Courtney was out the door, "Come on," she called to us, "we don't want to be late. All the good stuff will be gone."

I threw a jacket on Cait and headed out to warm up the car. It was a rare, cloudless November day. I soaked up Courtney's excitement and readied myself to hunt for winter treasures.

We were met by an already packed parking lot. Courtney wasn't amused when I said, "I think they cheated and came early."

Once out of the car we pushed through the doublewide doors and made our way to the small school gym. I held onto Cait's hand tightly and turned toward her sister. "Listen, Court," as I pointed to Cait, "you can't window shop. Let's get what you need and get out of here."

Courtney rolled her eyes and headed for the skis section. As I watched her walk away, my heart tugged. Our family called her their 4-H girl. While her long chestnut hair and well-defined features made her pretty, it was her rose-colored skin and dark, dancing eyes that gave her a wholesome, fresh glow. She was socially adept from the time she could crawl and her energy was almost always directed in positive ways. These two sisters couldn't have been more different. I understood her frustration with Cait that day. I felt it, too.

Cait was already attempting to escape from my grip as we moved through the narrow path to a table where Courtney was selecting a pair of ski boots.

"Those look nice. Why don't you try them on?" Courtney removed one shoe and pulled up her pant leg. Wobbling on the other leg, she slipped her free foot into the boot. I knelt down to help with the buckles.

"Don't forget you'll be wearing these with heavy…" I never got to finish my sentence. Cait was off in another direction. I got up, but not without stumbling over the other ski boot. *Damn.* I righted myself and slid between a parent with her two school-aged children next to us. "Sorry." The word dangled in my wake. I pushed past several other families, knocking into a rack with poles. I caught sight of Cait's blond head moving toward bright-colored skis. "Oh no you don't." From behind, I scooped her up just as she grabbed a blue one.

"Let me go," she tried wiggling out of my grip like an eel.

"This is Courtney's day. You need to be good." I knew my words fell on little deaf ears.

With Cait in my arms, I took a deep breath and went back to the boots, but Courtney had left them and was moving over to another table filled with skates.

"What happened to the boots?"

"Too big." Her eyes refused to meet mine.

"Don't you want to keep looking?"

She finally lifted her head away from the skates to look at us. "They don't have my size. We should have gotten here before all the good ones were gone."

By then Cait was crying. "Come on Caity, a little while longer." I felt myself beginning to break out into a cold sweat though the gym was cool. I didn't have the luxury of time to remove my jacket.

As we rummaged through the mountain of skates hoping for better luck, we eyed the ones we had dropped off earlier in the day being tried on by another young girl. I heard Courtney mutter under her breath, "At least she found a perfect pair."

It made us more desperate. I glanced along the table. Most of the skates were pretty beat up and looked either too big or too small. I wanted to head her back over to the boots. I was sure we'd find her something, but Cait's grunts were becoming increasingly louder as she tried pushing off me to edge herself out of my hold.

"Hey, you need poles right?" Before I had even finished my sentence, Courtney headed in that direction. I started to follow her when I heard a loud piercing yell from the child in my arms. I bent to put Cait back down just as she melted into a furry of cries and rants kicking and screaming as she met the floor. Her face was red and tear streaked. The noisy, crowded gym quieted to find the source of the commotion. I looked over at Courtney holding a pole under her arm to check its height.

I called over, "I'm sorry. We need to get out of here."

She glared at me, furious.

"Now, Court!" My angry words spat back at her. It wasn't her fault, or mine, or even her sister's, but I couldn't expect Courtney to understand. I was drowning in guilt.

I lifted Cait up in my arms. Shoppers hurried to clear a path for us to the exit. Cait wouldn't stop shouting even after we were outside in the fresh air and sunshine. It took all the strength I had left to get her buckled into her car seat. When I fell back behind the steering wheel, Courtney wouldn't look over at me, but I could tell her eyes were brimming with tears. Her words were muffled, "I hate her."

"Oh Court," I sighed, "You don't hate her."

I knew the challenges that came with raising Cait, and so did her sister. Lately, it seemed Courtney was on the short end of things, and as the sole parent, I couldn't fix it. If I went to watch Courtney's basketball game, I always ended up leaving the bleachers to wait in the gym corridor while Cait ran up and down. If we went clothes shopping, most of the time was taken up chasing after Cait who loved disappearing inside the racks of blouses and pants. We had stopped having fun.

I started the car and began the drive back home. Cait's cries had turned themselves into little whimpers. "I'm sorry about the ski sale, Court. There'll be others."

"No, there won't."

I could have argued the point or tried to explain away Cait's meltdowns, but I didn't. Instead, we drove the rest of the way in silence.

4

ISLAND GIRL

Cait and I sat together on the wooden bench built into the ship's stern. High above us, behind the glass window covered in sea spray, sat the captain, who expertly shifted direction to the east. At age five, this was Cait's first boat adventure. It was late summer. The soft wind off the water helped settle her. She nestled herself into me, pulling her sweatshirt's hood over her head. Every so often she'd peek out. When land began to take shape in the distance, we got up and walked to the railing, rocking side-to-side along with the boat. Holding on, we peered down at the white caps topping each small wave. Once the gulls appeared overhead, Cait gained her footing and pulled away to look up and return their shrill cries, giggling the whole while. I knew the ocean world would capture her fancy.

Our trip on the water was compliments of my friend, Jodi, who had extended an invitation to her family's island home for the weekend. With Courtney away at camp, I decided to invite along Evan, a fellow I occasionally dated, who knew my friend. Jodi, a potter, often had Cait visit her studio back home. Cait loved nothing better than to move the cool, damp clay through her fingers and make shapes that Jodi would glaze and fire—we called them Cait's works of art.

It was late in the afternoon when we arrived. As we maneuvered our bags down the gangplank, I got my first good glimpse of Cuttyhunk, one of the Elizabethan Islands off the Massachusetts coast. As soon as I saw Jodi and her husband, Jack, pull up in a golf cart to collect us, I was hooked on the place. There were only a few cars; visitors and islanders walked or traveled in old, recycled golf-mobiles. It was charming.

After dinner all the adults and Cait strolled past the one-room schoolhouse and white clapboard church until we reached the island's highest point, where we could see the sunset. I watched barefooted Cait balance herself on a flat stonewall holding my friend Jodi's hand. Her shoulders relaxed as she began to dance along, for once, sure of her footing. In the sun's magical afterglow, I could imagine Cait as an island girl, free to run wild among the things she loved. I felt comforted to think a place like this could exist just for her. It seemed to settle me, too, and I was able to tuck away the constant worry that at any moment Cait would unravel. I knew inviting Evan would make me especially vigilant, but here things seemed different. I wanted to believe that the ocean surrounding us helped insulate Cait from the world that often confused and frustrated her. That night the rhythmic call of the foghorn lulled me to sleep. I had forgotten that it was meant to warn sailors of unsuspecting trouble ahead.

Early in the morning before breakfast, Jodi took Cait and me to explore the rocks with their hidden tide pools. "Look!" There was a shriek from Cait as she held up a starfish and waved it in the air. There wasn't a squeamish bone in Cait's body as she fearlessly dipped her hand through the cold water picking up seaweed and hermit crabs. The pools were like Cait's private aquariums. Only the growl of hunger in her tummy could pull her away.

Later, we combed the beach for colored sea glass and perfect, smooth stones. Evan laid down the book he was reading to join us. Our voices and laughter mingled with the sounds of the waves as they rolled in. When we got back, Jodi gave Cait an old, oversized Cuttyhunk sweatshirt left by a past visitor. In the evening she sat with its huge arms wrapped around her while she rested her head on the back of the couch and contentedly stared out at the water.

On our last day, Jack took Evan surfcasting. Toting buckets and blankets, we followed the men through the worn sandy path lined with wild seafoam roses. It was an ideal spot to explore the tidal pools and sunbathe on a spit of sandy beach, but the whole time Cait kept a steely eye on the men as they repeatedly cast their lines into the water. "I got something!" Evan's pole was arched high in the waves as a fish flailed on the end of his line.

Cait scrambled over the rocks before the rest of us could reach him. "Put it in here!" She offered her pail as Evan, on the water's edge, played tug-of-war with his catch.

Only after seeing the frantic look on her face did it occur to me that Cait desperately wanted this fish. With it came a sense of dread in the pit of my stomach. After a short struggle, Evan finally reeled it on to shore. His prize was huge. He held it up laughing so I could snap a picture.

At the same time, Cait kept jumping up trying to grab at the fish, just out of her reach. "Put it in the bucket," she continued to cry.

Evan stepped away, "Stop it, Cait." His voice was firm. I sensed his growing impatience as he bent over it with his back facing Cait. "I'm returning the fish to the ocean." With that, he skillfully removed the hook and released it into the waves.

"Nooooooooo," Cait wailed.

Everyone gathered along the rocky shore that afternoon knew that fishing was a sport, except my daughter. She fully expected we'd be taking home our catch. As soon as it hit the surf, she threw herself down onto the ground and cried hysterically.

I knelt down beside her. "Cait, aren't you happy the fish gets to go back home?" Nothing I said consoled her. I finally reached my arms under her shoulders and lifted her up.

"We're heading back," I called out to no one in particular, and with that I dragged a struggling Cait off the beach. Out of the corner of my eye, I saw Evan turn away to cast another line.

Jodi followed us and put her hand on my shoulder. "Oh, Lyn." I was grateful it was Jodi next to me. I felt shaken and embarrassed. I knew not everyone on the beach understood Cait's behavior. It left me uncomfortable, and like Cait, out of place. Evan's annoyance stung.

Back on the path, Cait's sobs finally lessened. She pulled away from us and walked ahead. The winding path's subtle scent of roses and salt water had a calming effect. I was grateful to the island once again. As we continued our trek towards the house, with Cait clutching the bucket to her chest, I impulsively held up my camera and snapped her picture.

Months later while on a trip to the Netherlands, Evan purchased a pair of Dutch wooden shoes for Cait—perhaps amends for that afternoon on the rocks. It was a kind gesture, but it couldn't erase his reaction that day, or the way it had made me feel.

Cait and I have explored lots of beaches since Cuttyhunk. I like to think that her love of the ocean began there. She still can spend countless hours searching for treasures washed up on shore. Her room holds jars of opaque glass and shell fragments, smoothed and polished by the sea.

Although years have passed, whenever I look at the picture, it's hard to connect it with the scene that had transpired moments earlier. Instead, I choose to remember the innocent image of an island girl, on a sandy path, under an azure blue sky.

5

A IS FOR ASPERGER'S

Once Cait entered kindergarten I no longer had to worry if she'd be accepted into a program. This was public education, which meant all shapes, sizes, and behaviors. They had to take her, right? She already had her own small entourage: two speech and language pathologists, an occupational therapist, and an Essential Early Education case manager. Now it was just a matter of shifting over their services. I was hoping the transition would be seamless.

Weeks earlier I had received a surprise phone call.

"Hello, Lyn? Meg Kelleher, Cait's kindergarten teacher for this coming fall. I was hoping to arrange a visit to introduce myself."

"That would be lovely." It would, wouldn't it? A familiar face would help ease first day jitters. I was hoping it would do the same for Meg.

One late August afternoon, her car pulled into our driveway. Before Cait and I were down the steps, she was already dragging out her large satchel. Petite, with shoulder length dark hair and straight bangs across her brow, she appeared young and no more than a schoolgirl herself. As she walked across the gravel, she spotted

Cait and broke into a brilliant smile. In a moment she was kneeling down, eye-level, and holding out her hand. Cait took it in her own and grinned back. This woman knows her kids.

Cait didn't hesitate, "What's in the bag?" Her eyes and ears were all for Meg as she followed her and the canvas tote back into the house. Meg quickly positioned herself next to Cait at our dining room table and chattered about summer. Cait's barely audible one-word answers didn't deter her new teacher. To Cait's delight, she began pulling out her goodies. She first unearthed a colorfully illustrated book. She read it to Cait who was practically sitting in her lap by now. Paper and crayons came next. Cait took the cue and began her best rendition of stick people. Her usual fidgety behavior disappeared, and in its place sat a five-year-old, engrossed in making art. Meg and I discussed the coming year over her head.

"It looks like you love teaching this age group."

She smiled, "It's an exciting time for my students. I love to watch them joining letter sounds and reading for the first time, and then taking those same letters to begin writing their own stories." It was hard not to get swept up by Meg's enthusiasm.

But if Cait's new teacher felt some security that first day of school because she had met all her charges earlier, I knew better. My little, wide-eyed girl, sitting at the dining room table that late summer day, was not who she seemed to be. I wondered how long their "honeymoon" would last. A day? Five minutes? Everything kindergarten required, Cait didn't have. I had her preschool traveling-notebook to prove it. I already knew that circle time could send Cait into a tailspin. It wasn't just sitting for more than five minutes in one place. If a classmate happened to lean too close, he might be setting himself up for a slug in the arm. I imagined Meg's students reporting home to their parents about the girl who needed extra wide spaces on all four sides. Fine motor tasks, like cutting and gluing, were Cait's nemesis. She'd melt as soon as someone got out the scissors. Using glue led to the violent shaking of a hand until it spun like Linda Blair's head in the *Exorcist*. A demon? No, tacky fingers. Any direction with more than two steps was likely to get ignored. If verbal demands came too quickly, or the conversations were too loud, Cait would stop, drop, and roll, while kicking and screaming. What stoked Cait's fire? Her bottomless pit of frustration. Though eventually extinguished, the other children would fear her next episode. It was nothing they'd ever witnessed on Sesame Street. I was having a hard time seeing Meg's image of Cait, a child sitting still long enough to connect a letter to a sound, but I had no problem visualizing Cait's unsettling first days and their toll on Meg Kelleher.

It didn't stop me from cheering her on, "I'm amazed you can take the time to visit everyone."

She laughed, "I love the opportunity to meet my students at their homes. I learn so much."

I almost gulped out loud. If you only knew. Besides the acquisition of new skills, kindergarten was all about cooperative play and learning to listen—neither of which were easy for my daughter.

Turning to admire Cait's drawing Meg went on, "It gives me a chance to establish a relationship with both parent and student."

I had to admit I was impressed with her dedication, not to mention the spell she cast on my daughter. I put my misgivings aside. After Meg left, I decided I liked Cait's new teacher. I liked her a lot.

One afternoon in late fall, I arrived home to a blinking red light on my message machine. "Lyn, can you call me as soon as you get in? Thanks." Meg's voice with her home number equaled trouble. I felt my stomach lurch.

I flashed back to other times in Cait's short life when I had received similar calls from after-school programs or summer camps. The voice on the other end was always the same, "Sorry, it isn't working."

As I punched in Meg's number, I wondered if a five-year-old could legally be expelled from a public school. Meg immediately picked up. Her next words completely caught me by surprise.

"Lyn, I feel awful having to share this. I crossed a line today concerning Cait."

Was this a confession? "Meg, please, it's alright. What happened?"

"I've never done anything like this before."

I could tell at this point she was working very hard not to cry.

"Cait was having difficulty in line and wouldn't listen. She wouldn't look at me. Without thinking I tapped the side of her face in an effort to get her attention."

That's it? That's why you're crying?

"I touched her harder than I should have. It all happened so quickly. I crossed the line. I'm horrified."

No, you're human. I attempted to reassure her, not unlike all the times Cait's service providers had reassured me. "Meg, I completely understand. I know things like that can happen without thinking. I know you're upset, but really, it's okay."

Little did she know the wave of relief that washed over me. What I really wanted to say was, "All is forgiven. Just keep her in your classroom." No one knew Meg's own frustration better than I. Cait stretched this poor woman's patience to the brink that day. What happened didn't change my opinion of Meg Kelleher. She was learning her own new set of ABCs this year, along with the rest of us.

Despite my worst fears, Cait's early kindergarten days grew into weeks, then months, and through it all, Cait made steady, albeit slow progress. With the guidance of an extra adult in the room, she learned to manage circle time, and develop her early cutting and pasting skills. But whenever one task was about to be mastered, another challenge would take its place. From the start, numbers eluded her, and associating letter sounds to the words on a page made little sense, and writing them even less. Her teachers gave her a steady sensory diet, which even included the firm "brushing" of her torso, followed by joint compressions. Amazingly, it had a calming effect. Her language improved slowly, though her frustration still caused her to lash out. The notebook continued to travel, making its way home each night, sharing Cait's ups and downs. Meg still cheered her on, supporting each baby step.

Regardless of Cait's challenges, I knew she was eventually going to have to graduate kindergarten to make it to college. Wasn't I entitled to every parent's dream, even when the odds started stacking up against her very early in the game? I braced myself for the beginning of a long, long journey to Cait's university degree.

To my delight, when June rolled around, she did graduate. The ceremony was celebrated with white T-shirts that classmates signed, paper mortar boards with tassels, and rolled up diplomas tied with a bow. My parents drove up from New York. I wanted all of us to witness at least one march to pomp and circumstance.

Years later, I ran into Meg at a wedding. We hugged like old friends, sharing a special bond born the day she drove up our driveway and cemented months later with one soft tap.

6

ONE-CHILD CRIME WAVE

Cait loved the water. Summers I'd take her to our town's local beach. I always timed it after the morning swim lessons were over and the ropes taken down. As soon as we'd arrive, Cait was off and running with her net and bucket. As I spread our blanket, she'd be knee deep at the edge of the shore swooping down on some unsuspecting fish.

On one particular day it was packed. There wasn't a visible cloud in the sky and the air had a sultry summer feel to it. Kids were everywhere as families lingered to enjoy a perfect beach day. I walked Cait over to the dock and sat with my feet skimming the water's surface. She dashed after a bunch of rambunctious school-aged boys. Though just four, I could tell she desperately wanted to join the boy's fun. Every time they propelled themselves off the dock and sent out a big splash, she'd screech with laughter.

Somewhere in all the commotion Cait swung herself around and pushed a girl, younger than herself, into the water, giggling the whole while.

The young girl's mother and older sister were wading inches away. "Oh my God!" the mother screamed.

I jumped up from where I was sitting and caught up to them just as the mom grabbed her youngest by the arms.

I think it was the panic on her mother's face that made her daughter begin to wail. That just fueled the mother's open contempt for Cait.

"I'm so sorry," I shouted from behind.

The victim's mother looked around and unfurled her fury, "That child has the devil in her!"

She stormed past the other swimmers with her arms locked around her toddler, while daughter number two trailed behind. My eyes followed them back to their towels. I wanted to make her take back those words, but had no ready reply. Instead, I turned to Cait.

"You can't just push people off the dock!" Only crazy people do that!

From the short wooden pier Cait looked down at me. "Sorry." The word was no sooner out of her mouth and she turned to run off again.

"Cait, stop!" In her moment of hesitation, I hoisted myself back onto the hot pier and grabbed her. I forced her down into my lap before she had a chance to cause any more catastrophes. My heart was pounding. I should have gone with Cait to apologize, but I was too pissed off. How dare the woman imply that Cait was evil? Cait was possessed all right, but it was her inability to control her impulses that held her. When she was little, I never knew what random object she would suddenly grab to throw or put in her mouth. As she got older, I wasn't able to gage how she would react to a situation or, like that day at the beach, to someone innocently standing next to her. The truth, if I were honest, was every time I tried getting inside Cait's head, I'd secretly beg the same question: What possesses you?

We sat there for a while, watching schools of small minnows dart under the dock each time a swimmer came too close. Cait's blond hair felt warm and downy underneath my chin. As I looked down at her Little Mermaid swimsuit and small toes splashing in the water, I contemplated her most recent action: the near drowning of a three-year-old. I no longer took comfort in her surface innocence, but was left to wonder, What next?

With Cait, I never had to wait long.

Although my children were born and raised in New England, I was a New York City girl. My parents, then both in their seventies, continued to live in the house where I grew up, on the outskirts of Queens. Now a parent myself, I could appreciate their very different parenting styles.

At age fourteen, my dad had traveled an ocean by himself, from Eastern Europe to the US, to join his father, who was already here. My mom, on the other hand, was born in the States, with close family not more than thirty minutes in any direction. I often reflected that it couldn't have been easy for my dad, who almost raised himself. His reward was an unrelenting work ethic that followed him even after retirement. He loved being busy and always had something to repair. Though my dad was the most generous man I knew, on the surface he was gruff and didn't tolerate poor behavior. I watched him struggle trying to understand Cait. My mother was my "go-to" parent. She was good-natured, with a soft spot for her younger granddaughter. Cait knew the difference between her two grandparents. While she adored my mother, she held my father at a distance.

A couple of months after Cait's beach crime we were at my parents' house, getting ready to depart after a visit.

"Are you positively sure you've got everything?" My mom stood in the kitchen as I made my fourth trip outside to the car.

"I'm sure," but I told Courtney to go upstairs and double check. Cait had gotten up later than the rest of us, so I promised I'd bring her favorite cereal on the ride. My dad had left for a doctor's appointment, undoubtedly relieved to miss our hectic exit.

"I don't want your stinky cereal," Cait began her departure complaints.

"You sure got up on the wrong side of the bed this morning," I joked pouring the Cheerios into a plastic container.

"I'm not eating it!"

"Look, we're already running late. What's wrong with this cereal?" I already had started pleading.

"I refuse!" A new vocabulary word for Cait. I didn't know whether to applaud or cry. Before I could decide, she was out the door, slamming it with a force that belied her mere fifty pounds. One of the glass panes shattered.

"Holy crap," I looked at my mother.

"Oh my, thank God your father's not here."

On the other side of the door I could hear Cait sobbing. She ran down the porch steps.

"You better bring her inside," my mom's voice was near panic.

At the same time, Courtney raced into the kitchen, "Wow, she really did it this time."

I was tempted to let Cait run all the way home to Vermont, but instead I rushed out to where she stood on the walk and grabbed hold of her hand.

"Come on, Cait." She wouldn't look up or stop crying, but took my hand and followed me. Her small body shuddered with each new sob as we neared the door. We stepped over the glass, but once inside she pulled away and ran into the living room.

I sank into a chair at the kitchen table.

"I can't believe this. Mom, I'm really sorry. When Dad comes home, he's going to be pissed."

My mother slid into the chair next to me holding a dustpan and broom. "I'll take care of your father. Replacing the glass will give him something to do this afternoon."

We looked at each other and laughed.

After I helped her sweep away the remnants of Cait's ill-placed temper, my mom went to work her magic. It brought me back to the blow up arguments I used to have with my dad as a teen. It would always play out the same. I'd race to my room slamming the door and minutes later I'd hear my mom, the peacekeeper, knock.

I heard their muffled voices in the next room occasionally interrupted by a deep exhale from Cait as her tears began to subside. When I walked in, Cait was awkwardly cradled in my mom's arms as she rocked her.

"Please don't slam things, Cait. Look at what can happen. Your Papa will fix the glass."

Now calm, Cait promised she wouldn't.

Though I didn't want to admit it, I knew there were times I was more like my dad, struggling to understand my daughter, responding to her poor choices with knee-jerk reactions. Right then, I wanted just an ounce of my mom's patience and wisdom. Once, she told me that there would come a day when my daughter would be a comfort to me. I laughed, telling her I couldn't imagine it. But deep down, I wanted to believe her. And just like her, I wanted to believe in Cait.

7

CAMP GRANADA
(Hello Muddah, Hello Faddah)

The summer Cait turned six, I made plans to attend a summer workshop so I signed her up for a nature camp conveniently located on my school's grounds. That way, I'd be only a short distance away if there were problems. I filled out the camp questionnaire, identifying all of Cait's special needs. I had no idea how they structured their program, but I hoped for the best. In my heart, I knew it was a long shot.

It rained the first day, but that didn't deter Cait. She was ready and waiting for me at the door with her rubber boots and favorite purple-fringed umbrella. I had a good feeling.

As I was taking notes in the back of a classroom that morning, I felt a presence behind me. A six-foot fellow, half hidden under his hooded rain slicker, loomed in the doorway, water dripping off him onto the carpeted floor. He looked directly at me. I got up quietly and followed him into the hall. Cait stood between us dwarfed by his size. I lifted my gaze to meet his as he shared his concerns. "She seems to be having a hard time."

"Hard how?" I needed to know.

"She's been struggling to follow along with the activities, but mostly she wants to do her own thing."

"Do you know the reason?" I regretted my words even before they were out of my mouth. Could he know how ridiculous my question was? I'd been having Cait tested since she turned three.

"Early in the day things seemed calmer, but, we're concerned that this afternoon will be more difficult for her. Maybe we should try just mornings."

"No problem." But it was a problem. Now I would need to attend the workshop, while supervising my daughter.

Still, I felt like I needed to reassure him. "We'll see you in the morning," I said. "Hey, maybe the sun will be shining by then." As if that would help.

"She's a really cute kid." He started to walk away, leaving me with the cute kid. "The staff hopes we can make it work."

Cait fiddled with her lunch bag.

"Come on, let's see what games and books I can round up while I'm at my class."

The sun did shine for the next few days, but not on me. Mark, the tall young man in charge of Cait's group, worked hard to include her as best he could, but things didn't improve. If they played predator/ prey, she was adamant about being the predator. If they were doing leaf rubbings, she'd insist on using the bug microscope. Coaxing Cait to do what the other kids were doing took time from the rest of the group. Before lunch each day, she was back with me in the hallway playing with her books and toys alone.

On Friday I thanked Mark. We both agreed to end her camp experience after that first week.

"Maybe next year," he said. He sounded so optimistic, now that she was leaving his charge.

"Yes, I'm sure we'll try it again." I could be optimistic, too.

I did try, again and again, until Cait reached her teens. Each time I asked myself, "Why send her?" Was I simply being too thickheaded or dim witted to see the obvious? Or was I after a family album with happy camper photos. Why did I work with such blind determination to give Cait experiences like her peers? Truthfully, it was the hope that maybe the experience would make her more like her peers. I wanted her to join in and have fun doing the things other campers enjoyed doing. I wanted her to belong.

Early each spring, over the next seven years, Cait gave me silent permission to plan her summer camp adventure. I'd always talk it up and show her lots of pictures of laughing campers with friendly counselors. She'd usually shrug and agree to go, probably to get me off her back. But I appreciated her willingness to "do time."

Each camp had a slightly different offering than the others. We tried day and overnight camps, Girl Scouts and the YMCA, but the outcome was always the same. I figured that Girl Scouts were all about confidence and leadership building, so imagine what they could do with my daughter. That dream ended at 9:00 a.m., after only four days in the program, with another week left to go.

The following summer, we tried a YMCA camp for boys and girls. I hoped that Cait's energy would be less noticeable if boisterous boys surrounded her. Sadly it was her grumpiness and lack of compliance that stood out. She was only a couple of days into that camp when I heard from their nurse. After a short discussion about meds, she got to the main point of her call. "She's a wonderful girl," she shared, "but there's too much going on here for Cait."

Each time I collected her from another camp, the counselors were eager to say how much they enjoyed getting to know my daughter. But they were quick to add that a shortened stay might be best.

Cait and I soon had our end-of-camp conversation down pat.

"So what did you like best?" I'd ask.

"Free time."

"Really? Why's that?"

"It's quiet and I can read alone on my bunk."

Cait just didn't fit the camper mold. She wasn't the enthusiastic, campfire-song-singing participant most camps preferred. Since Cait was still working on sustaining a give-and-take conversation for more than five minutes, she'd never make a summer camp friendship that would last a lifetime. I knew many programs tried to instill confidence. Their formula didn't work for Cait. Her counselors were always a bit teary and full of hugs when I'd pick her up, calling out their good-byes and good-lucks as I drove off with a quiet and relieved Cait beside me. For what it cost, I could have taken deluxe summer vacations in the Caribbean and whiled away the hours on hammocks in the sun. But I was determined to succeed.

During Cait's camp career, I did find two programs tailored to her needs, both extremely expensive. I decided it was time to pull out the big guns: my parents. Luckily, my folks were more than willing to help their struggling granddaughter.

One camp I found in upstate New York catered to campers with challenges similar to Cait's. When we arrived, we dropped off all her meds with full disclosure. At the time, Cait was taking varying doses of Ritalin throughout the day to heighten her attention span and Celexa to ward off her grumpy moods. The Ritalin came with side effects, which included tic-like behaviors such as throat clearing or nose twitching. If this happened at camp, we'd need to change her dose. I was a bundle of nerves driving back home that afternoon. But during her few phone calls home, Cait always seemed cheerful. When her counselor got on the line, she assured me everything was fine.

Cait even managed to deal with the camp's two-day, overnight canoe trip. She shared that the other girls from her cabin spent the whole time complaining about bugs and how tired they were.

"And you didn't?"

"Of course not. We cooked over a campfire. It was great!"

For the first time since Cait started going to camp, I hung up smiling.

The next summer we decided to try another camp that was private, but close by. It had a maximum of three campers to a tent. With such a small charge, Kyla, her counselor, figured Cait out in record time. "She's our animal girl!"

The camp had pens with rabbits and goats that campers could feed. Cait was right on it. Kyla also signed her up for individual sports like tennis and fishing. Cait was happy, and if there were bumps along the way, I never heard about them. She stayed for the full three and a half weeks.

I will never know if the camp experiences bolstered Cait's confidence, widened her world, or molded her into a law-abiding citizen. But the camp photos in our family album show her tanned and smiling. In the end, maybe an exotic island for the two of us wouldn't have been nearly as good.

8

SQUARE PEG

I hated school pictures. Every September when the envelope marked "Picture Form" made its way home in the bottom of Cait's backpack however, I'd fill it out anyway, checking off "Package F," the cheapest, offering just one five-by-eight and several tiny wallet-sized images. I hoped the photo company, and anyone else who glanced at the order, wouldn't think my meager choice was a reflection of how I felt about my daughter or an indication that I didn't want to mark her elementary school years. To me, their photographs looked stilted and unnatural, while I saw Cait as spontaneous and alive. Still, I looked forward to the class shot that accompanied every package. Cait was always seated up front, and through photographic magic, appeared poised and happy. I'd scan the group and note with pride that she was as cute and appealing as her peers, especially with her toothless grin in first grade. She blended in with the rest of her classmates. There were no telltale differences. Yet, that quick snapshot didn't tell the real story that lurked behind the picture of the square-peg girl who was anything but a perfect fit.

When Cait began her elementary journey, I began my own. Faced with twelve long years, stretching ahead like the Great Wall of China,

I refused to consider any path but the one that led straight to a college gate, where after four more years she would be prepared to make her own way in the world. My biggest fear was that Cait wouldn't fit that model, that she would change the trajectory. What scared me the most was not being able to predict where she'd land. My fears propelled my vigilance each step along the way.

At the end of kindergarten, when Cait was assigned to Liz Davenport's first-grade class, I immediately questioned her kindergarten teacher Meg's placement decision. "I know Liz," I said, trying not to whine. "I'm not sure if she's the right fit for Cait." If people could be described as dog types, then Liz was a Jack Russell terrier: small in statue, with a commanding bark, bottomless energy, and unrelenting determination. I knew Liz professionally and respected her many talents. She was everything Meg said she was, but I also knew the single-mindedness that allowed her to get so many things done, would clash with Cait's own. If that weren't enough, the school had combined the first and second grades, so if Cait and Liz butted heads, it would be a long two years. "Liz is talented and experienced. She'll be great." Meg wouldn't be deterred.

The other teacher who taught first and second grade was nearing retirement. I wasn't sure if Meg was protecting her senior colleague from the challenges that came with inheriting my daughter, or if she was determined that her kindergarten graduate would have continuity. Yet, parents don't get to pick their children's teachers. "I trust your judgment, Meg." I gulped, swallowing what would be the first of many doubts.

Meg's initial intuition about Liz proved right. She loved big themes, and so did Cait. Though Cait's budding work habits were riddled with her willful and inattentive trademark, she sponged up everything her new teacher had to offer. The afternoon I visited their open house, Cait shuffled her way over to me wearing an oversized, pink Mandarin gown and clutching a paper parasol. It was the culmination of their China unit. "You're here!" She grabbed my hand and pulled me toward the hanging paper lanterns and dragon kites. Despite her fine motor challenges, her slightly lopsided dragon waved in the gentle breeze of the open hallway along with the rest of them.

"Cait, these are amazing."

"I know," she cried, jumping up and grabbing at her kite's red-ribbon tail, almost tearing it from its honored place among the others.

Before I had a chance to look more closely, I was getting pulled over to the display table. I could tell it was like a delectable buffet to Cait; she was uncertain what to gobble up first. She toyed the hand-made abacuses and grabbed the chopsticks to deliver a solo drum performance on the table's edge. "Put those down," I whispered, glancing with envy at the parents and children calmly sharing their work. Cait was like a Chinese firecracker, snapping and crackling. She raced around the room with me in her wake, barely keeping up.

Finally, Liz called the children up front to sing. I sank into the nearest chair and began praying. I was learning to fear the worst. Would she throw a fit? Or stand in the middle of twenty-one other Asian-costumed children with arms folded, refusing to participate? I wondered if any other parents were having similar images. When I noticed the educational assistant edging her way into Cait's line of vision, I began to breathe a little easier. Whatever telepathic powers she possessed, they seemed to have a calming effect on my daughter.

As soon as the performance ended, I headed directly to Liz, "This was wonderful! Thanks so much for all your hard work." She exchanged a knowing grin. While parents lingered, I found Cait back at the chopsticks ready to drum out another set. I bribed her with a special dessert waiting at home, not wanting to end the evening with an outburst. Though Cait had on her picture-perfect pose, I knew her overly excited state usually heralded a tantrum. We were out the door by the count of three.

A month later, while seated around the table with Cait's team, I got my first insight into how challenging my daughter was for Liz. We had started a series of blind medication trials in the hope of addressing attention issues. The most recent consensus among the team was that Cait had attention-deficit/hyperactivity disorder—ADHD. The psychologist had some suggestions for other ways to target Cait's oppositional impulses that were surfacing as well. He turned to Liz. "I want you to use a stopwatch." I glanced over just as Liz rolled her eyes. "Add up the times she shows resistance to a direction, or is off task, and take that time away from something she finds pleasurable."

I felt Liz's pain. It was a record-keeping nightmare, not to mention it resembled a puppy-training class. Pretty soon they'd be parceling out kibbles for good behavior. I wasn't any more comfortable than Liz with his suggestions, but then she shocked me. "Sometimes, I think Cait easily fatigues, and it's what leads to some of her inappropriate behaviors. Maybe we need is to consider shortening her day."

I shot up in my seat. Was she crazy? It was my turn to cringe. I worked full time and was having enough difficulty managing after-school care. Cait had already been expelled from the understaffed afterschool program for her unpredictable behaviors. Now Liz was suggesting we decrease her school time. Maybe if I had had the funds to hire a private nanny I would have entertained her ideas, but I didn't.

Liz eventually bought into the stopwatch suggestion and relegated the bookkeeping to Cait's assistant with some success. Happily, her shortened-day idea was forgotten.

Weeks later I ran into the assistant while shopping at our local market. Her two sons attended the same school. Perhaps it was this familiarity that propelled her to speak candidly with me. "Lyn, I need to share something. I want you to know Cait and I are out in the hall *a lot*."

Her emphasis on the last two words got me. She didn't need to say more. I knew Cait didn't always cooperate. She could easily be over stimulated and act out. If an activity was too noisy, learning was difficult. But I got the feeling Cait was relegated to the desk outside the classroom a significant part of her day. More than that, Cait was on display for the rest of the world to see. I was furious with Liz. I'd be in the kitchen washing dishes and catch my reflection in the window rehearsing what I'd say to her, or in the car, practicing my airtight case to an invisible passenger. Each time I'd end with the same closing argument. So why is Cait in the hall, Liz? And don't tell me it's quieter. Quieter for whom? In addition to everything else my daughter had going against her, there was now another item to add to the list: the label "hallway" kid.

I did call Cait's school, but my well-practiced script was with Shannon, the school guidance counselor, who was sworn to secrecy. "Shannon, it's come to my attention that Cait seems to be getting most of her work done outside the classroom these days." I had made the decision not to get into it with Liz. Within days, a "go-to" space for Cait was found.

Though I had concerns about the way Liz handled things, Cait learned. It was with Liz that she developed her powerful love of books. By the end of second grade she was a reader. Years later, I'd reflect on this strength of hers and acknowledge its roots could be traced back to Liz's class. But I also acknowledged that something else took root during those early elementary-school years: Cait's differences. Even a perfect classroom picture couldn't change that.

Three years later, I found myself trying to strike a bargain again, only this time it wasn't about where to send her. "Barbara, would you consider keeping Cait another year in fourth grade?" I had been agonizing over my conversation with her fourth-grade teacher for weeks. I knew there was a stigma attached to retention, but would it matter to a girl who was socially disconnected?

"Wow, that's a hard one, Lyn. She's with such a great group of kids, and overall, her academics are okay. We tend not to retain students unless there are some very strong reasons to justify it."

"Do you really see her holding her own with sixth graders next year?" It was a combined fifth- and sixth-grade class. I had struggled from the start wanting Cait to fit in, but her immaturity was beginning to stand out like a beacon. While her peers were talking about clothes and music, Cait was still playing with beanie babies and dinosaurs. I needed to buy her time.

Barbara realized it, too. "I'll bring it up to the administration. It's a team decision. We can discuss it further at our next meeting.

As I left her classroom that day, I spotted Cait in art, flanked by two familiar girls from her class. I could hear them instructing her. "Take this pencil, it works better."

"Look at this picture, Cait." One girl showed her something she'd drawn. A peal of giggles emerged from their three bowed heads. I couldn't help but smile with them. One or two classmates still invited her to their birthday celebrations, but their roles were beginning to morph into guardians instead of friends. It bothered me that she didn't have play dates, but she seemed happy at home, left to amuse herself. When I looked at her moving along to the next class, I worried. I couldn't envision Cait being able to hold her own surrounded by pubescent, preadolescent sixth graders, even with the supportive class I was now asking her to leave behind.

Later in the spring, the team met again. True to her word, Barbara shared my concerns. "She's a late spring birthday, so that places her on the younger end of her class anyway." I didn't care how they justified it, as long as they agreed.

I felt some relief knowing that Terri, her assistant would stay behind, too. From New Jersey, she left a career in business to pursue her dream of living on a horse farm. The field of education was new to her. Short and stocky in stature, Terri wasn't much taller than Cait, yet her warmth and sense of humor were infectious. She and Cait immediately clicked over their mutual love of animals, but even better, Terri *got* my daughter. I believed it was her work with the free-spirited horses on her farm that enabled Terri to understand Cait on a different level than the rest of us did. She seemed to have a bottomless reserve of patience for a young student who showed little patience for anyone else.

I also learned that nothing comes without its price. While I adored Terri and her willingness to continue her work with my daughter, I worried about Cait's dependency on her. Occasionally, I'd show up for a meeting and glimpse the class walking through the hall with Terri walking alongside my daughter. Sometimes, Cait would reach out and take her hand. Can you help my daughter, but remain invisible while you do it? The roles that Cait's assistants played in her education would haunt me throughout her time in public school. While the one-on-one model helped Cait to navigate her studies and relationships, in some ways the assistant replaced the teacher. How could Cait become independent and capable, when she had a personal sentinel along the way? And how would others judge her?

Cait eventually moved into the fifth and sixth grade, rejoining some of her old classmates. Right before her exit from elementary school she was up for her three-year evaluation, to determine her continuing need for services. Once again I was uneasy. Cait's challenges didn't fit the mold of a typical reading or math disability. Hers was more complicated. Her difficulties communicating with peers and her lack of social awareness and maturity were becoming more pronounced—and middle school was all about peer relationships. Despite her average intelligence, Cait's inability to focus continued to follow her like a big cloud that rained down on her work habits and organizational skills. School would continue to place difficult demands on Cait and me. At times it felt like a crazy roller-coaster ride. I desperately wanted to shut my eyes, but I knew I needed to keep them open if I wanted to see what was coming up next. Besides, you don't get off a roller coaster when you're climbing the next big hill.

When the evaluation was complete and the team reconvened, it was determined that Cait fit the Asperger profile. Though Asperger's was a rare diagnosis at the time, especially for females, we had always believed that Cait had a type of communication disorder. Her long-standing social imperceptions made the new diagnosis conclusive. Maybe all the dots were finally connected. I was relieved there would be no question about continued services as she moved ahead. But if I were honest with myself, the new nametag didn't really matter—

not unless it opened the door to an easy fix—and I had been on this journey long enough to know there was no such thing.

That spring, Cait, along with fellow sixth graders, performed Hamlet. She was cast as the second lady-in-waiting. To her delight, she got to dress-up in a purple velvet gown, with draping sleeves and tied bodice. Surprisingly, she executed her small part with perfection. But in typical Cait-fashion, she also knew all her class-mates' lines, including Hamlet's, and reminded them when they screwed up. As I sat in the audience on opening night, praying she'd stay in character until her curtain call, I remembered back to a prior performance and those earlier days with Liz. I wondered about my square peg. She had spent her fair share of time outside the box during her elementary school years: in the hallway, repeating a grade, on the sidelines apart from her peers, shadowed by adults with good intentions. As much as I appreciated everyone's efforts, could our Cait ever be reshaped into a perfect fit? Maybe she truly was a lady-in-waiting—waiting for the rest of us to acknowledge that not everyone is destined for a round hole.

9

THROUGH THE LOOKING GLASS

One of the challenges Cait and I faced was finding the right medications to help her pay attention in class and ease her sometimes-unpredictable behavior. Finding the ones that worked was mostly trial and error. Even now, when I think of all the tried and failed medications or doses, I can hear the Jefferson Airplane, with Grace Slick's iconic voice singing my version of a 60's lullaby. I imagine Cait drifting off, dreaming of mom's neon colored pills that made her smaller, and other times larger. It's the image I carried when I thought of those pills and their impact on my daughter.

While Cait's meds weren't hallucinogenic, I had had her popping pills since the first grade. I didn't feel good about what I was asking my six-year-old to ingest, but my dreams of ivy-covered university walls wouldn't come true if her behavior kept her in the hallway.

When a school evaluation first suggested attention deficit disorder with hyperactivity, I immediately conferred with Cait's doctor, Susan, and asked about medication. I liked Susan and would have followed any advice or prescriptions she offered. She was the one who provided the article on autism and informed me Cait didn't fit the profile.

"When I'm considering medication for any child with symptoms like Cait's, I prefer approaching it by conducting a blind trial first."

"Blind trial?" It sounded like one more evaluation. I wanted to help my daughter right now.

"Over the next six weeks we'll try Ritalin, but in two different doses, and during that time we'll also have her take a placebo."

"You mean a sugar pill?"

"Exactly. You and the school will need to fill out a weekly check-list so we can get an unbiased account from both home and school." It sounded like Cait was about to embark on a new version of show-and-tell: Can you guess what pill I'm on?

I appreciated the careful tactic Susan was using to make sure this was right for Cait. At the same time, I groaned inwardly at the thought of informing Cait's first-grade teacher, Liz, that she'd have yet another form to fill out, but I was sure she'd love the thought of a compliant and easier charge.

Cait's doctor went over it again. "Two different doses and a placebo. Two weeks on each. After all the checklists are sent in, I'll look them over and decide where we go from here."

I didn't know whether to thank her or cry. "Great. See you in six weeks."

It didn't take long to guess when Cait was taking the placebo. It came down to figuring out the right dose of Ritalin.

When Cait finally started her daily Ritalin regime, I had a hard time wrapping around the idea that she was now taking a stimulant when she was already charged. As it turned out, the parts of Cait's brain that influenced her attention and impulse control were actually under aroused. Ritalin affected the natural chemicals in Cait's brain, increasing the dopamine signaling, which helped her brain cells to communicate. Deep down I knew there was no magic bullet to change Cait's world, and that it would take more than one small pill to move her along in life. It was just one piece, albeit an important one during her school day. But it didn't come without a price: side effects.

Her new medication affected appetite. Cait was never a big eater. I worried that her already slight frame would get even smaller. We tried to work the dosage after mealtimes, but with enough time to "kick in" before her next activity. Still, at each well-child doctor visit, she hovered around the twenty-fifth percentile on her growth chart. Though Cait never complained about other side effects, like headaches or upset stomachs, she did experience rebound. When the medicine would start to wear off, Cait's behavior would quickly deteriorate and her hyperactivity would return, sometimes worse than it had been before the dose. It was her rebounds I found the most difficult.

I spotted Jean, the afterschool program's leader, at a picnic bench, pouring apple cider from a large gallon container into small cups, as her charges gathered around her. A young mother, she had recently started a new afterschool program. The air had the chill of late fall, but it was still nice enough for the children to sit outside and enjoy their snack in the last light of day. Bundled in sweaters and jackets, most of their heads were bowed as they munched on cheese and crackers. As I walked closer to the group, I silently admired Jean's beautiful sweater. Oversized and knit in earth tones, it was clearly homespun wool and undoubtedly crafted by Jean, herself. Cait, now seven, had informed me that Jean owned chickens and goats and asked if we could as well. Though I wasn't ready for a barnyard family, I did appreciate Jean's gentle approach with the children and assumed she'd be a good fit for Cait.

As I approached the group, I could "feel" Cait before catching a glimpse of her. A flurry of energy was coming from her side of the table. I caught sight of her blonde head and red-and-white, striped sweater. She was flicking a cracker crumb onto the grass, followed by another and another.

"Cait, cut it out," complained the girl to her right, but Cait continued without looking in the girl's direction.

Only when she saw me, did she stop. "Mommy!" She ran over and grabbed onto my waist and hung there. "Mommy, Mommy, Mommy!" she laughed and then released her hold, running back to the table and grabbing her cup and another cracker.

Jean turned from the bench looking a little frazzled. "Lyn, hi."
She walked over. "Could we talk for a minute?"

When she was out of earshot from the group, I knew exactly
what she was going to tell me.

"This situation isn't working for Cait. She has a lot of trouble
listening and is constantly getting into the other children's personal
space. She's a sweet little girl, but I have to think about what's best
for the other kids."

What could I say? I was hoping this young earth mother with her
own young children would embrace mine.

"Jean, I'm sorry you feel that way." My feathers were ruffled.
Sorry Cait's not your perfect crunchy granola kid. But whom was
I kidding? Cait was difficult, and why should she single-handedly
make afternoons difficult for everyone else.

"I'll need at least until the end of the week to make other
arrangements."

"Of course."

I hadn't a clue what those other arrangements would be. What
I did know was that Cait was on her Ritalin rebound. The end of
her day was never easy. She was tired and spent, and when we added
rebound to the mix, it spelled disaster. It made all her ADHD-like
symptoms worse. I would have added a third pill for after school,
but that would have kept her up at night.

I walked back to where Cait was sitting and had her follow me
to where the pieces of cracker were scattered. "Cait, you can't just
throw food like that." Silently, the two of us knelt down and picked
the crumbs off the grass.

Rebound didn't just occur at the end of the day, it happened
whenever Cait's dose was wearing out. When it did, her restless
behavior took a downward spiral. We were constantly returning to
the clinic, reporting why this dose wasn't working and checking out
other stimulants new to the market.

We moved from our pediatrician to a psychiatrist, now overseeing
this part of Cait's medical care. In the process, we met some amaz-

ing doctors. I appreciated their thoroughness as they interviewed me, Cait, and her teachers, always carefully checking for weight and sleep loss before making any adjustments. I thought of them as pharmaceutical angels watching over us. It still felt, however, like we went through stimulants the way Imelda Marcos went through shoes. Drugs like Adderall, Concerta, Focalin, Vyvanse, and even a skin patch lined our shelf. Our medicine cabinet looked like the pharmacist's station at CVS. Cait stayed on some of these drugs for years before something more effective replaced them. The most significant improvement in Cait's drug regimen was time-release tablets. They allowed Cait to skip the nurse at lunchtime, but even better, they reduced the effects of rebound. Yet, I discovered that when we ducked one side effect, there was always another to take its place.

The year Cait turned thirteen, the two of us drove down to Ocracoke Island off North Carolina for April break. Ever since her Cuttyhunk days, she, like her mother, loved the beach and finding treasures. Long road trips for her were always easy as she could read for hours barely coming up for air. I had always wondered how anyone with attention issues like Cait's could bury herself in a book, but she did.

"Ahem."

I glanced over. "You okay?"

"Yeah."

Two seconds later. "Ahem. Ahem."

"You're not okay. What's wrong?"

"Nothing!"

By the time I got on the New Jersey Turnpike, I thought some alien, meant to torture me for every wrongdoing I had ever committed, had replaced my daughter. Every mile she was clearing her throat.

"Oh my God, Cait. Can't you stop it?"

"Stop what?" And then she'd do it again.

I played the radio as loud as I dared to block it out. How could I have not noticed before the trip? Maybe it had to do with sixteen hours of close quarters. Finally, we got to our destination. The island seemed to ease her tic-like throat clearing. It was less pronounced on the ride back, but still there—there until another tic replaced it.

Cait's tics were always morphing from things like throat clearing, to facial twitches, to picking at her skin. Her back has scars from her reaching around and jabbing at any little pimple she suspected under the surface. Even now as a young adult, she takes tetracycline, an anti-inflammatory medicine to counter the damage, and she keeps her nails short. In the middle of her worst tic episodes, we tried a non-stimulant med, Strattera, which worked on increasing a different brain chemical than the stimulant family of meds, but it didn't work for Cait, so we were back on the stimulants, hoping the tics wouldn't come back.

Just as Cait was reaching her teens, her psychiatrist added Lexapro to her daily med regime. An antidepressant, it had the added benefit of offsetting irritability. It countered the grumpiness that often cropped up in part due to the stimulant. If someone accidently bumped into her, her response was to swing around and accuse them of pushing her. "What do you think you're doing!"

It didn't help her social status, but I knew in the end no med was going to single-handedly improve her judgment. The only one who could do that was Cait.

On weekends and during the summer, Cait continued with the same dose as during the week. I reasoned it would be unfair for Cait to operate in her restless mode for two days and then go back to her drug-induced norm. She never really said anything to me about how she felt on or off her meds. I just assumed, when my little Mexican jumping bean was at rest, she was better off. I would soon find out I was mistaken

For years, Cait went along to her older sister's riding lessons. While Courtney trained, Cait was occupied by the endless supply of cats, dogs, and a potbellied pig that roamed around the funky old farmhouse where Kim and Kelly lived and gave riding lessons. When Courtney stopped to go away to college, Cait took her place on the saddle.

Watching Cait, I never dreamed that she'd graduate from the lunge line that tethered her to her instructor in the middle of the rink. As the horse and Cait went in circles, Cait was forced to listen and perform each direction called out, sometimes standing in her stirrups, with her hands stretched out or on top of her head, practicing her balance. She finally became untethered, and soon after, was jumping over wooden cavalletti poles, which Kim or Kelly had strategically placed around the rink. When her instructors raised the poles, I held my breath, secretly amazed. Both women were tough on Cait, but Cait responded. Riding was like a sensory buffet to all her systems. While she mastered posting to her horse's rhythm, she still loved letting herself be jolted up and down, laughing the whole time.

One day, while waiting for Cait in the barn, Kim turned to me. "Lyn, we've a horse show coming up in a couple of weeks. Nothing fancy. I think Cait's ready to join us for this one." Kim turned back to help Cait hang up the saddle. "Right, Cait?"

"Sure." It didn't sound like much of a commitment on Cait's end, but when they tried encouraging her the year before, she had flatly refused. I was thrilled. We had a navy jacket and tall black boots, hand-me-downs, sitting in the back of Cait's closet just waiting.

As we were leaving the barn, Kim made a surprise request. "Can you skip the Ritalin that day?"

I thought I had heard her wrong. "Skip it?" Had she taken leave of her senses?

One Saturday morning, a few weeks earlier, we had rushed out of the house forgetting Cait's meds. I remember profusely apologizing, worried that her focus would be off.

Kim's voice brought me back. "Don't give her the meds. She's so much better without them."

"Are you serious, Kim?"

"When she's not on them, she's in tune with herself and the horse. Sure, she's a little more distracted and points out every butterfly that crosses her path, but she's Cait. It's beautiful to watch her connect with her animal."

She didn't need to say anything more. "Okay, we'll skip the Ritalin."

"Great."

As Cait and I drove home, I wondered about what we had been missing out on all these years? I knew that in a classroom, Cait needed help paying attention, but the world wasn't always a classroom. Maybe the occasional distraction wasn't a bad thing. In my eager attempts to help Cait experience success, I had failed to ask her how she felt.

Kim was right. Cait gave a flawless performance on her horse that day. Unlike *Alice in Wonderland*, there wasn't a "magic" cake waiting for her. On her own, without her twentieth-century potions, Cait rode like she was ten-feet tall.

10

FANGS AND FEATHERS

Thanksgiving dinners were at our house. The four-and-a-half-hour drive to my parents in New York at Christmas was challenging enough. Thanksgiving travel easily doubled the traffic and time, so that holiday we reserved and celebrated at home. Our table now included Cait's stepsister, Sam, two years her junior, and her step-dad, Mike, along with various friends who found themselves like us wanting to avoid hours in a car.

Staying in Vermont also meant casual dress, but not for Cait. One particular year as we sat down and clasped hands to say grace, I couldn't help but glance across the table at her instead. Perfectly erect in her chair, she wore a fringed suede vest with her hair tightly pulled back into a single, long braid. Two eagle feathers stuck up behind her head, while peacock feathers dangled, one from each ear. She looked both regal and whimsical. No one murmured a word about this year's attire. It was, after all, Thanksgiving. If I had been a stranger to the group, the only thing that might have tipped me off to the eccentric nature of this lone Native American girl with uncommonly blue eyes and fair hair was her age. Most eighteen-year-olds wouldn't have been caught dead in anything as crazy as Cait's getup, but then you don't know my daughter.

Cait's love of dressing up started at an early age. I found it curious that though she struggled with sensory stimulants, like loud noises and bright lights, she didn't fit the Asperger mold when it came to touch. Most Asperger children avoid scratchy textures and often dress in comfortable sweats. For Cait, nothing was too lacy, frilly or tight fitting. She adored being noticed.

At age four, she decided to have a hand in her own fashion wear. With permanent magic markers, she gave herself a tattoo look all over her naked body. It took two solid weeks of daily bathing for the last of her signature designs to wash off. Halloween was her favorite holiday. She'd continue to wear each costume long after the last of the candy was gone. Sometimes they were even her substitute for pajamas.

In fifth grade, Cait and her stepsister inherited a treasure trove of costumes that a friend's daughter had outgrown. Their favorite was a matching set of Bavarian miniskirts and puffy blouses. Cait wore hers with red fishnet tights. She looked like a Paulie Girl filling beer steins for her rowdy patrons. I explained to the girls that under no circumstances were these particular outfits to make it onto their Halloween costume list. Although Sam was two years younger, her dress-up frenzy faded after the first couple of months, but Cait's was only getting started. A year later I discovered her Heidi costume in the bottom of her school backpack. I was horrified.

"Tell me you didn't put this on at school."

"Only after gym," she confessed, "but then I changed right back. I swear."

"Oh my God, Cait, this is going to get you into *big* trouble."

My reference to "big trouble" was our unspoken understanding that went something like, "Please don't alienate yourself from your classmates by doing something you'll live to regret."

Courtney and I were vigilant when it came to how Cait dressed. We were always trying to curb her natural penchant to stand out amongst the crowd. Courtney, who was closer in age to Cait, also feared embarrassment. Their disagreements about correct attire usually surfaced around sister outings.

"Cait, you are *so* not going out looking like that." Cait was in one of her frumpy moods. She walked downstairs with oversized camouflage pants held up with a large belt and alien-looking moon boots. Courtney blocked her way. "Change it."

Cait scowled, "Which part?"

"Seriously? All of it!" Courtney refused to allow even a little of her sister's quirkiness in public.

"Fine!" Cait swung around and stomped back up the stairs with her sister close behind. Courtney picked out what she felt bordered on reasonable and Cait acquiesced. She loved nothing better than to accompany her big sister into town and was not going to risk being left behind.

No one could escape Cait's unusual attire, including her stepdad, Mike. But unlike the rest of us, he never seemed to take notice. One time, when they were heading out to the movies, Cait walked into the living room adorned in all black, wearing bright red lipstick.

I cringed. "Absolutely not, Cait." I didn't want Mike to feel awkward in public with her.

"She looks fine." He never flinched.

"Thanks, Mike!" Cait turned away from him and shot me one of her "I told you so!" looks.

While she ran to her room to grab a jacket, Mike defended her right to dress the way she wanted. "You really need to lighten up and not always be on her case."

"Tell me she doesn't look like someone out of a second-rate vampire movie."

"Lots of kids dress like that." Mike taught high school. Maybe he knew more than I was giving him credit for, but he wasn't Cait's mom, and Sam, his daughter, never gave him one gray hair. My own head was full of them.

I decided to let it go. As my gothic star headed for the door, I gave her a hug. Deep down inside, I knew Mike was right.

It was impossible to raise Cait without appreciating her love for accessorizing, which, when she was young, revolved around hats.

For years, she wore different versions of English suede caps and Annie Hall felt fedoras. During the winter, she was always garbed in a faux-fur Russian style, with nothing but her nose sticking out. She also had a penchant for costume jewelry, especially large crosses adorned with fake rubies. Once, at an antique shop, she spent her last twelve dollars on a fireman's ring. She never seemed to choose anything that wasn't eclectic or different.

I was willing to acknowledge we had our very own fashionista. I did, however, have some boundaries I wasn't willing to cross.

"Got everything ready for school?" As I started the car, I glanced over at her. She was looking dead ahead, her thoughts elsewhere.

Right before we got there, I looked in her direction again. Something was off.

"Cait?"

"What?"

Why did she sound like she was sucking on marbles?

I entered the turnaround to drop her off.

"Should I meet you back here or at the town library?"

"Library."

She couldn't wrap her tongue around her Rs.

"Cait, look at me."

I caught sight of two slightly exposed fangs where her front molars should have been.

"Cait."

"I'm not wearing them to class. Honest."

Now I could see the full effect. I scanned her neckline for bite marks.

"Well in that case you won't mind handing them over so I can keep them in a safe place."

Cait was into her vampire craze well before the *Twilight* saga hit the big screen. This was the start of her Goth look. She reluctantly handed over the fangs. They were the expensive kind that you could mold onto your own teeth. To her delight, they looked authentic. I ended up tossing them in the trash the first chance I got, hoping it would put an end to her Dracula phase. It didn't.

For five years in a row she dressed up as a seductive vampire for Halloween: flashy black dress, long-hooded cloak, and tall black leather boots. Cait's appetite for fangs fueled her acquisition of endless pairs of pointy teeth. I could never be sure if she would show up to class with them, and I suspected the cloak was worn other than on its designated day.

Several years later I watched my daughter across our holiday table again. This year she had emerged in a long, pink silk skirt with an over layer of black taffeta that matched her seventies black silk blouse. Her slender frame and long, straight hair gave her a Hollywood glam effect. I couldn't deny there were times Cait possessed a flair others might envy. I also knew all those clothes came from our local thrift shop. I had to give her credit. She was by far the cheaper daughter to dress, and sometimes she hit the jackpot. But the next day she could as easily be back to wearing a pair of torn jeans, with a skull tee shirt and spiked choke collar. Whatever the outfit, I was learning to take a deep breath and embrace my daughter's unique sense of style. In my overly zealous attempts to right her world, I hadn't stopped to listen to what she had to say. The girl who struggled to find the right words to express herself, had found her voice when it came to what she wore. Everyday she was telling us a different story. So this Thanksgiving as we held hands to say grace, I knew I had a lot to be thankful for, even the occasional fang and feather.

Part II

DAMSEL IN DISTRESS

"…as your father, my instinct is to protect you…Other people will want to protect you too. But remember that you are not a damsel in distress, waiting for some prince to rescue you. Forget that prince. With your brain and your resourcefulness, you can rescue yourself."

Author Brad Meltzer, *Heroes for My Daughter*

11

KING ARTHUR'S TABLE
or The Art of the IEP

I wanted to believe that the teachers and support staff who planned Cait's school days and guided her growth experiences were like the fabled Knights of the Round Table. You know, the ones who flanked their king: each one honorable and good, and led by the most noble of them all, King Arthur. Whether or not Arthur was simply legend, we hold what he stood for in high esteem; creating equality and doing the right thing. In the world of special education this should mean making sure all students get the services and programs they need, no matter what the cost. Surely if a legendary king and group of knights could foster these guiding principles, there must be a similar group that can guide contemporary public schools.

I knew that our damsel, often in distress, was in want of an Arthur and a group of closely aligned professionals who'd provide a program that met her needs. Unfortunately, the countless tables at which I found myself seated in my years of parenting Cait were rarely round and the players not always knight material.

I had begun my table hopping when Cait was barely three, at my own dining room table. Cait's essential early ed team, Kelly and

Claire, gathered around as we attempted to untangle the mystery of her early language delay and other curious behaviors. I discovered my youngster's early toe walking meant something, and her ability to climb cabinets in order to reach a cookie wasn't necessarily an indicator that all her other motor skill acquisitions were in check. We started early intervention. Deep pressure massage to her arms and legs followed by compression of her joints relaxed Cait's overly sensitive system. It was my first introduction to a tactile diet. She loved to be sandwiched between the floor and a weighted beanbag or to maneuver her body through a narrow tunnel. It felt really good to have these two women on my team.

My next table wasn't a table at all, just chairs set up, semicircle in the hot, stuffy office above the classrooms of the daycare center where her teachers, speech and occupational therapists all suggested something more serious might be going on with Cait. But when I'd look at my bubbly three-year-old, I was left wondering. What are these overzealous people thinking? Still, I never doubted their caring instincts. Cait's services continued as she mastered using the toilet, sitting in a circle, and finding words to express herself.

Meetings at Cait's elementary school meant sitting low to the ground with doll-sized chairs. I respected any adult who could sit in one more than ten minutes. (Our meetings usually lasted an hour.) I found that her teachers and her new special education team were still fighting the good fight, figuring out who my little girl was and what types of help made the most sense. There were even Arthurian spies among the lot. If any of Cait's teachers had her working out in the hallway, it wasn't long before another team member made sure there was a more private space.

Specialists were brought in to test and assess. Suggestions were taken to heart. Cait continued to increase her use of language by adding new words to her growing vocabulary list and to fine-tune motor skills like writing her name and playing catch. There were occasions I'd hoped for more direct services by the professionals evaluating her; instead they passed off their recommendations to her current educational assistant to carry out. Still, I never doubted everyone had Cait's back and was working hard on her behalf.

At times, Cait's team felt like an extension of our own family. We even shared love notes. When Cait was in second grade, Mike and I started dating. He would woo me with silly, funny letters. One morning, while in a rush to fill Cait's backpack with some documents her case manager, Vicky, had sent home, I inadvertently picked up one of Mike's notes. There was a message from Vicky on my answering machine later that day. "Lyn, check out Cait's backpack for an envelope. You are one lucky woman. My husband never did that for me!"

Later when I looked, it was one of Mike's more evocative notes with computerized kisses along the border. Over the next several months, I couldn't sit across from Vicky at a meeting without turning red, but she'd just wink. The silly note seemed to make us more real to each other.

I ended up running into Vicky several times at the post office, where she'd talk to me about her own son, who she suspected was on the spectrum. She shared her worries, and in return, I'd offer up any new resources I found. Vicky was only a part-timer at Cait's school and managed a staggering caseload. I advocated increasing her hours to the school board, even when it fell on deaf ears. Cait needed more team members like Vicky, but for now I felt Cait was in safe hands until she moved down the road to middle school.

Communicating Cait's story to a new set of teachers was daunting when so much of her history was passed along orally and most things were learned by trial, error, and simply being around her. I understood I couldn't keep her in elementary school forever. We both needed to move up—Cait to seventh grade and me to my next table, larger than my last, with adult-sized chairs, and significantly more knights.

I assumed Cait's new Arthur, or learning specialist, would be the person delivering and coordinating services and holding everyone accountable. Above all else, this person would get to know the inner workings of my now pre-adolescent. But unlike Camelot, I soon discovered it didn't work that way.

Special ed at Cait's new school was synonymous with one name, Ann Wells. Though she was Cait's case manager for most of her time in middle and high school, Cait never once worked with her. Everything fell into the lap of the educational assistant hired to follow Cait to her classes. By the time Cait was a junior, and Ann was no longer at the high school, the same case-manager model was still in place, and regardless of my best efforts, I couldn't change it.

Fortunately for Cait, she had savvy assistants. If anything, case managers were great at hiring. The assistants were all very capable, and each was a believer in the abilities of my daughter, but none, except for Tate, Cait's eighth-grade assistant, fresh from Ameri-Corps, had a degree in special education. Interestingly, some of Cait's best test scores came under Tate's tutorage. She knew exactly how to prep her for a science test, assist her in math, and help her memorize a poem. After Tate's departure, I asked if we could access some of the computer programs Tate used with Cait. I was told to go find them myself. Wasn't that their job?

Cait no longer received direct services in speech and language, and occupational therapy, but specialists could consult with teachers, if the need arose. I knew that there was only so much time in the day, now that Cait was moving between classes. I wanted to believe that the intention was to manage Cait's time, not cheat her out of much needed help.

Cait's education plan included the direct teaching of social skills, in this case after school with Patrice. A high-school parent herself, Patrice had worked with several local programs to assist children who had developmental challenges. Her background was in the arts. She first noticed Cait when volunteering her talent in costume design for the sixth-grade play. Patrice was the donor of the costume box that had given Cait and Sam so many hours of pleasure. Her perceptions about Cait were uncanny. She was hired to meet with a small group of middle school girls. While the girls weren't especially athletic, and didn't participate in afterschool sports, they were all in need of varying degrees of social supports. The group, called Crafty Girls, was the brainchild of speech and language pathologist, Kathryn, who'd later lead Cait's social thinking group while she was in high school. Patrice worked on their communication and social skills through activities ranging from sewing and cooking, to field excursions into town and even a fashion show. The girls seemed to relish the group's camaraderie, and for Cait, it was her first opportunity to feel as though she belonged.

I feared middle school would be the scariest of times for Cait, but it wasn't. The fights I fought, like extra time on tests, were only skirmishes. I put away my sword and learned to accept that some of the challenges in Cait's world were beyond my control. So as I looked ahead to high school, I figured moving to the next grade would be no more intimidating than changing lockers.

Little did I know that I'd be slaying dragons.

12

BARKING DOGS

The walk between Cait's high school and the town library took no more than three minutes. The path from the hilltop campus to the small brick building on the town green led past two-hundred-year-old homes, with granite hitching posts still intact. As the late day sun streamed into the library, with its modest collection of books and art, the overstuffed chairs were warm and comfortable, beckoning patrons. The property sat on a grassy knoll with a large yard and picnic bench under tall sugar maples, which bordered the parking lot out back. The site rolled down to a brook lined with cattails and reeds, a perfect marsh for catching frogs. A wooden bridge allowed for easy crossing to another grassy hill, where the elementary school stood. It was an idyllic spot, a picturesque childhood scene filled with charm and a sense of town history, except for a group of rowdy boys.

As Cait walked alongside the road, after the last bell, weighted down with her heavy pack, she could hear the boys and their unified dog-like howls from a distance until the car they were driving approached and closely followed her quickened step. I used to imagine the noise at first made her jump, shattering a thought or daydream. I was convinced it became the reason she'd often choose to wait for me at her school most days. There I'd find her reading in the hallway with her back up against a hard wall. I was sad to think about her being deprived of the walk and the place she loved since her early elementary school days.

As her parent, I felt helpless. There was little I could do to stop them. No leash or threat of the pound would curtail a bunch of smart-aleck high-school boys, young pups really. There were days I was ready to tie them up to the nearest tree. I'm sure their wolf calls happened more times than Cait was willing to admit. She didn't know their names, though they made it a point of knowing hers.

"They bark at me from their car as they drive by," she'd complain, only when she was in a sharing mood. If I probed too much, she'd just shut down.

"You need to tell Mr. Miller." The dean was coach to several school sports teams, and beloved by everyone. No matter how much cajoling I did to try and get Cait to advocate for herself, she shied away, or told me what I wanted to hear. "I've told Mr. Miller. He knows about it."

"Is he doing something?"

No answer.

Bullying wasn't new to Cait, but it was to me. When I first became privy to the inner workings of her daily life, I was indignant, but sadly, in some ways, immobilized like my own daughter. The offenses were always subtle, under the radar, too quick to catch, but nonetheless, crept their way into my daughter's days.

Once, while at Cait's school, I passed the dean's office and saw him sitting behind his desk. I knocked and stuck my head in without waiting for an invitation.

"Mr. Miller, Cait mentioned some difficulty she's having with a few boys after school. They've taken to heckling her when she's walking to the library."

"Have Cait come see me. We'll find out who's behind it."

I never felt reassured that Cait's complaints about anonymous hooting from a runaway car amounted to a real offense in the school's book of wrongdoings. The dean was a nice man and fair on the playing field, but I doubted that he "got" my daughter. So when I dropped her off most mornings, I'd usually call out before the slam of the car door, "I'll meet you later. Right here!" She'd look up and give a nod. We conspired in silence. I, too, came to accept the safer of the two after-school alternatives and hoped the roar of the janitor's vacuum was enough of a threat to any wayward, straggling boy-pups left behind.

13

MOM, THE DRAGON SLAYER

I probably sat around five different tables during the time Cait was in high school. The most formal was in a small room next to the school library. The table, wide and long, practically filled the entire space. It was by far the most intimidating. If all of Cait's teachers and team members showed up, we had to squeeze in, but that was rarely the case. The day I met Aubrey Banks was a "half-table" meeting.

Most of us were clustered at one end, when I spotted an unfamiliar face sitting alone at the far end, opposite us. I figured she was our new LEA—the town appointed educational representative who was charged with approving or denying district funding. In our town the job belonged to the principal of the elementary school. Up to this point it had been Chip Wheeler, the principal while Cait had attended school there. Unlike Chip's countrified demeanor, Aubrey donned short, platinum hair that was stylishly cut. The business suit she wore clinched her air of authority.

I stood up and walked over. "Hi. We haven't met. I'm Cait's mom." I was about to extend my hand, when her body language told me not to bother.

"Aubrey Banks," and with that, she looked away.

I went back to my seat, and peeked a glance at the others sitting next to me. Everyone's eyes were averted. I didn't need ESP to pick up on the negative vibes Aubrey Banks sent out, or that the team had a closet full of issues with her.

The tenor of our meetings was about to drastically change. Chip rarely showed up for meetings. He had faith in the case managers and believed that any request for funds would be reasonable and necessary. Then Chip retired. In his place came Aubrey. No two people could have been more different. If Chip had been cast as Arthur, then Aubrey was none other than Morgan le Fay, Arthur's evil half-sister.

Aubrey wasted little time and whipped out her notebook. Her questions felt like sharp-edged daggers with perfect aim.

"Explain exactly what type of after-school program Cait is currently participating in?"

"How many hours of direct support is she receiving in each class?"

"I'm noting that she's down for a counseling session once a month. Doesn't the district have access to its own counselor?"

I audibly gulped at the last one. Her therapist, Jane, a developmental psychologist, had joined the team right after Cait was diagnosed with Asperger's. Familiar with this relatively new disorder, Jane jumped onboard, eager to support her new patient. Jane had been seeing Cait for the last five years. Did Aubrey seriously think I'd consider switching to someone new? My insurance paid for most of it. Her suggestion would save the district a few measly dollars.

The entire time she interrogated the team, she carried an aura of impatience, like a royal scepter. It seemed to be directed at all of us, but I felt it most. She never once looked me in the eye. I figured out pretty quickly I'd be in for some major battles, though I wasn't yet clear whose blood and how much of it would be shed. However, one thing was crystal clear. From this point forward, I needed to be Cait's Arthur.

When Cait moved up to high school there were some changes: the biggest one was the block schedule. The theory behind it was fewer, but longer classes each semester, allowing time for greater depth and opportunities for project learning. Great in theory, but years with Cait taught me not every student would benefit from extended class time. Different minds processed and learned differently, and Cait's was definitely different. The high school argued it was ideal for someone with organizational challenges like Cait: three or four classes to juggle instead of six. But they failed to take into account the attention factor. Cait couldn't sustain focus for more than thirty minutes on a good day. Now they'd just tripled the time. True, if she was interested, she could stay on task all day, but that was usually relegated to computer games and the occasional five-hundred-page Harry Potter book, started in the morning and finished by sunset.

On top of placing a new demand on her attention, there was the issue of condensing a year's worth of information into half the time. While it may work in a history class, algebra and Spanish were different stories. I realized high school was going to have a whole new set of challenges.

Most special needs students on an individualized plan have one or two meetings a year to evaluate and then plan the following year's goals. Cait averaged five or six. At the start of each term, it was to introduce Cait and her plan to a new set of teachers, and then a few more to check in and adjust her program if needed. Anyone on the team, including me, could call a meeting if a concern cropped up. Aubrey attended all of them. I was always tempted to turn and ask, "Aubrey, don't you have better things to do right now, like running the school down the hill?"

Aubrey saw Cait through dollar signs. You would have thought the coffers were in her pockets. I could foresee more battles on the horizon, with Aubrey holding the purse strings.

I needed an ally at those meetings—someone smart and perceptive to watch Cait's back, so I turned to Jane. I sometimes compared Jane and me to a Mutt and Jeff duo. I'm tall and given to rambling when expressing my concerns over Cait. Jane's small in stature and a good listener. Her quick wit and depth of knowledge about the developing mind helped her come across as cool and collected. While I held up my parental end, which could be emotional at times, Jane balanced me by being factual and direct. She knew the nature of the beast and how to attack it. On the day I had my Aubrey blow up she was there.

We were tucked into a room the size of a walk-in closet. At the start of meetings we always did a check-in, updating each other as to Cait's progress. I found it hard to control my foot tapping during those times, wanting to get on to the more important stuff. Recently, our meetings had boiled down to math, where Cait was struggling. Right after the last person gave their update I announced my concern. "I'm worried about math. Cait can't manage it in a block schedule."

Jane followed my lead, "It seems like we keep going around and around on this with no resolution or plan in place."

I kept the conversation going, "We need a different kind of math model for Cait. She needs a certain number of math credits to graduate."

"When the information is too rapid, it's confusing and it makes accessing it at a later date extremely difficult." Jane now had everyone nodding in agreement.

We piggybacked each other perfectly, never missing a beat until Aubrey broke her silence. "Why are you worrying about math when Cait doesn't even know when she's smiling."

We all veered our heads in the direction of the cutting remark. I wasn't the only one stunned. She might as well have called my child a drooling idiot. Aubrey tried to bury her hideous comment with an avalanche of words. "I know a parent who is also a math consultant. I'd like to invite her to assess Cait's current math function and give a recommendation on where we might go from here."

All I could do was stare at her. Let's see if Ms. Aubrey Banks knows when I'm frowning.

As the meeting ended and people began leaving, I held back. Just before she stepped out, I called out after her, "Aubrey, can we talk a minute?"

She turned to face me as I stood up. Jane had stayed seated next to me. In as even a voice as I could manage I asked, "What exactly did you mean by 'Cait doesn't even know when she's smiling'?"

"I can't understand why you're worrying about math when there are other issues."

I felt the color in my cheeks reddening and my voice rising, "For your information, Aubrey, Cait most certainly knows when or if she's smiling."

From the corner of my eye I saw Jane was standing now too. She only reached my shoulder, but her stance was that of a prizefighter who'd just entered a heavyweight ring. I was remotely aware of the door to our closet-like room being closed, as our heated voices were now audible to everyone outside its walls.

Jane took over and gave Aubrey a crash course in Asperger's 101.

"Cait is building greater awareness of her frustration level and learning to temper her reactions. This doesn't equate with a total lack of emotional awareness."

"Aubrey, Cait is bright, but struggles in math." I was pissed. "That's a separate issue. How dare you imply my daughter shouldn't receive the tutorial help she needs because you think she doesn't know when she's smiling."

Aubrey was smart enough to know when to back down. We exited the room still in one piece. But for me, it wasn't without renewed determination. I needed to impale this woman the only way I knew how. Permanently remove her from Cait's team.

I made my appointment with the superintendent's office and stated my long list of complaints. Aubrey's exit from the team was faster than I'd thought. I don't think I was the first who had issues with her administrative style. Unfortunately, I soon discovered she wasn't the only dragon that needed slaying.

14

BABY FACE NELSON

C_{ait} is a collector. When she was young, her treasure hunts often yielded a tossed gum wrapper, lost earring, broken barrette, or plastic gem off the top of a ten-cent ring; anything that shined or caught her fancy would make its way into her pocket. I learned to check her clothes carefully before tossing them in the wash. Her collectables were saved in special boxes or simply arranged along her windowsill. If I suggested the trash as a good place for some of her finds, I was met with a definitive "No" and a roll of the eyes suggesting I simply didn't appreciate their value. I sometimes joked that in her past life she must have been a raven, since they shared her love of shiny objects. Cait was flattered.

As she grew older, her tendencies for acquiring goods grew as well. At a young age she stole candy off a shelf from our local gas station. I doubt it was her raven eye as much as her sweet tooth. My own eagle gaze caught sight of the wrapper as soon as we got into the car. I had her march back in to return it and apologize. The girl at the register hid her smile as she looked down at this towheaded, wide-eyed urchin and accepted Cait's admission of guilt. I was convinced the embarrassment of the act would be enough to steer her away from a life of crime. It wasn't.

From the elementary school playground, Cait moved to middle and high school classrooms and corridors. In middle school, she continued to collect "Cait style": a canvas painting rejected by a classmate in art, an interesting slab of wood from the scrap barrel in shop class. I appreciated her spirit of reusing and recycling, but soon my earlier worries began to resurface. One day I eyed a glass beaker from science sticking out of her backpack, and several days later, I cringed when I discovered the soft velvet Elizabethan head-dress from theater class.

Cait had been working in the drama room as part of her after-school, Crafty Girl group. Crafty Girl took on new meaning. I immediately contacted Patrice. She went with Cait to return it the next day. The drama teacher had taught Cait and knew her love for eclectic styles. She accepted her apology, but with a stern reprimand. I, too, appreciated Cait's love of fantasy and escape. I understood her coveting the crown and could see her crowned and waiting for her pretend prince. But my dream was soon replaced with Cait behind bars wearing an orange jumpsuit.

"I swear, the next time you steal something you're going to end up at a detention center or worse—jail!"

"Sorry, I didn't mean to," she whispered. It was another one of her meek apologies.

"Explain how taking something and stuffing it into your pack is not meaning to!" She didn't grow up in a den of thieves. Where was this coming from? I was fast becoming the parent who's never more than a step away from losing it.

Just a week later she went on an after-school outing with Patrice to a funky secondhand thrift shop a couple of towns away. A used, unpaid for, video made it into her bag. Cait reasoned I'd balk at another film with her shelf already full of them, but she didn't predict my reaction in regard to another theft. Maybe she was banking on my not noticing, but Patrice did. Cait had to return to the store with the owed money and watch as I re-donated the film. I was pissed. No child of mine was landing in Sing Sing.

I knew that justice had to be swift and scary. At work the following day, while I was still reeling over the tape heist, I approached

Paula, a coworker. Paula had four grown sons and one was employed in law enforcement. Steve worked with kids as part of the local drug prevention program. He was young, handsome, and personable. Maybe I needed a brash, Al Pacino look-a-like, but Steve had known Cait from infancy. I shared my daughter's crimes with Paula and begged her to call him.

I rarely find myself at police stations and the day we drove into the parking lot, I suspected Cait was feeling as queasy as I was. When I glanced over, she was stone faced and quiet. At least she wasn't crying or attempting to jump out of the car window, so my chances of getting her into the building were good.

When I entered, the sea of guns and blue made me feel immediately guilty, even though I'd invited myself in. If I took a lie detector test, buzzers would have sounded off like crazy, but my only criminal act was motherhood.

Steve ushered us into a conference room. He sat across from Cait, appearing very official, but the calm demeanor in his voice seemed to put my petty-theft criminal at ease "So Cait, do you know why you're here?"

"I think so." It was barely above a whisper.

"Why don't you tell me what you think?"

Cait proceeded to fess up.

"What you've done is stealing. It doesn't matter how small or incidental, it's taking something that's not yours."

Cait nodded slowly.

"And stealing is breaking the law." Accenting the last word, he clinched it. "Let me show you what happens when you break the law." He got up. Cait's eyes grew to the size of two silver dollars. I could have bowed down and kissed Steve's feet. He succeeded in doing what I, her mother, was never able to do, scare the crap out of her—and it got even better.

Steve led us down a long hallway. "Here's the holding tank, Cait. This is where you have to spend a night when you're first arrested."

Cait turned mute and stared. It was a closet-sized space with only a single hard bench, barely big enough to lie on. I hoped her imagination was running rampant.

From there Steve took us to two cells, side-by-side. The cramped, uncomfortable space, with no privacy, was more than enough to steer anyone away from a life of crime, but the real clincher were the bent bars in one of the cells.

Cait suddenly found her voice. "Look at the bars, what happened here?"

"An angry occupant." It was all Steve had to say.

Cait's expression spoke for her—"I don't want to be here with a crazy person!" By the time our tour ended, Cait was two shades paler than when we had walked in. I felt like I had won my case and didn't even need a closing argument.

On the ride home I wondered about Cait and her own moral development. I knew that all kids told lies at some point, but stealing? I could reason that deceit was in many ways at the core of our human nature. Didn't the caveman hide his meat so as not to have it taken away? And if he found his neighbor's, wouldn't he sneak off with it when times were lean. Basic instinct, but I knew Cait had sophisticated intelligence, way beyond cavemen. She'd eventually get it. And she did. Although I had to admit, I watched her like a hawk every time we went into a jewelry store to make sure she had outgrown her raven tendencies.

For that moment, my little Baby Face Nelson had come to the end of that trail at least. What I didn't know then were just how many episodes in Cait's life had a way of resurfacing and morphing into something new.

15

BEEN THERE, DONE THAT

Late one evening at around 8:30, the phone rang. My father was now in his eighties so I steeled myself for bad news. The voice on the other end surprised me. "Hi, Lyn. This is Nan, the school nurse at the high school. I hope I'm not calling you at a bad time."

I immediately assumed Cait's school supply of meds had run out. "Hi, Nan, you're not interrupting anything." As I assured her, my mind was racing. How quickly could I get her a refill? I'll need to apologize in writing for being so forgetful.

"Lyn, this is a little awkward, but I need to follow up on an accusation Cait made today."

Not the meds. But if it's not the meds, then what? My antennas went up trying to follow what she was saying. Accusation? Bullying? Was someone tormenting Cait again?

She cleared her throat, "Cait came to school upset today. She confided to one of her teachers in the learning center that you hit her."

"What?" I was thunderstruck. I, mother of the year—no make that almost two decades—was being accused of child abuse? My mind raced through that morning, and I suddenly found myself with a pit in my stomach the size of the Grand Canyon. I was guilty as charged. I could see it now, Child Services knocking at my door, Cait following them down the steps, suitcases in tow, and an ever so slight smirk on her face. Well, wait until she finds out that the overcrowded foster-care home will not only forget to send her meds to school, they won't bother to check her homework. She'll become a high school dropout, living on the streets before she reaches her senior year.

"Lyn?"

I found my voice. "Nan, let me explain exactly what *did* happen this morning."

Parenting Cait wasn't easy and I was no saint. While friends and family would commend me on my patience and perseverance, I secretly knew they hadn't a clue about its price or what happened when I was running on empty. What they assumed to be virtuous persistence was more like blind ambition. I was driven beyond all reason. My Cait must experience success in high school and have the opportunity to move forward with her education. I knew she was bright and loved learning, just in her own way. It always boiled down to the "square peg in the round hole" syndrome, and sometimes it was painful for both of us. It ended up with me pushing, pulling, and filling in where services or help were lacking. I discovered that accommodations on her individual plan were often just words on a printed page. They allowed her extra time on tests, but the workload was always the same. What might take another student one hour to accomplish, might take Cait three hours. Modification of the assignment never seemed to happen. And how could I have her accept less when I wanted her to move onto higher learning with her peers? We had to keep plugging away. Evenings were never pretty. The evening before the school nurse called was no exception.

"Cait is everything done for tomorrow?" The TV was too loud for her to catch the question. "Cait, turn it down." No response. I pressed mute. Her eyes never left the animation playing across the screen. I turned it off and she finally looked up. "Cait, are you done with homework?"

"Yes."

"Are you sure about that?"

She stood up. "I'm really tired," and with that she headed up the stairs.

I would have been willing to bet a week's salary that no one in her high school class went to bed as early as she did. Sometimes, the light was already out in her room by 7:30 and she hadn't even said, "Good night." I understood that managing a day at high school was exhausting for her. It was like a hiker climbing the trail with one leg. Everyday she was being asked to make her mind work differently from how it was wired.

As I gathered up her books and papers into a pile so she wouldn't forget them the next day, her assignment sheet stared back at me. The homework she had started, but not finished, was due, in its entirety, tomorrow. How could she just conveniently forget or shrug it off? I didn't care if she was in sleep mode; it needed to get done. I headed up the stairs. Crap, I'm dreading this.

"Cait?" I pushed her door open.

"What now?" she moaned, half asleep.

"You're not done."

"I'm sleeping. Leave me alone."

I turned all the lights on in her room.

"You're getting up and finishing this." I had the assignment in my hand. "You blew it off, Cait. You can't just leave it unfinished."

She threw off her covers, "Fine!" and stomped down the stairs.

I followed two steps behind. "Let me help."

"NO, I'll do it myself." Her eyes welled up, but no tear fell. "Leave me alone!"

"Okay." I left to let her work though it herself.

An hour later I was back, ready to try again. She was still only halfway through. It was already 10:00 p.m. and I wanted the evening to end. "I know you're not happy about this but neither am I."

She wouldn't make eye contact.

My own exhaustion was turning into anger. "This is your own doing and I'm tired of picking up the slack." I lifted the laptop off the table and walked over to the couch. "Just dictate. I'll type."

"Fine!"

It was grueling. "Cait, you've four more questions to answer. Come on."

I had to dig deep for each word that came out of her. "Because why Cait? He wants you to explain it, you know, like . . ." I knew more of my own words were being spread across the page than should have been, but I didn't care. Who should I be angrier with, Cait or her teachers?

I finally turned toward her, "I'm done. This is crazy, just go to bed." I shut the laptop screen, and with that she ran up the stairs and matched my frustration by slamming her bedroom door behind her.

A restless night's sleep didn't do much to alleviate either of our moods the next morning. While she sat at the breakfast table, I asked if she had a plan for how she was going to finish the assignment. She shrugged. I walked over to where she was sitting and lightly cuffed the back of her head. "Wake up, Cait. This is supposed to be your work and your responsibility." She fled from the table screaming in her wake, "I hate you! Just leave me alone!" I sank down in the chair she had just nearly knocked over. I knew there was no time to reason with her.

Neither of us said a word as I dropped her off that morning. It took the twenty-minute drive to my own school to shake off some of the weight of Cait and her assignments. Those nights always left me feeling guilty. Was I asking too much? Should I let it go and not care? I knew that would be asking the impossible of myself, but was I in turn seeking the impossible from her? Sometimes, to fall asleep at night, instead of counting sheep, I counted down semesters until Cait would graduate.

Like most blowups with Cait, the storm passed and when I picked her up at the end of the day, all remnants of our earlier argument were gone.

"How was your day?"

"Great. In science Mr. W. brought in a new bearded dragon. It's awesome. We should get one."

That afternoon I found her working in her room with her schoolbooks opened. Was it my imagination, or had she seemed more compliant and gotten down to her homework right away without even a reminder. Maybe she was feeling guilty over slacking off, or she was more motivated than I had given her credit. Nan's call came several hours later.

After I hung up the phone with Nan, I walked back into the family room. I was somewhere between mortified and appalled. "Cait, that was the school nurse who just called me."

"What for?" She looked as clueless as I had ten minutes earlier.

"It appears she needed to investigate an accusation you made today that I torment you and smack you around."

"Oh, my God!" Cait looked genuinely horrified. How quickly she'd forgotten her own part in this.

"More like 'Oh, my God what the heck did you say to them?' "

"I was angry with you." At least she wasn't denying it.

"How did I *hit* you, Cait?"

"It was a Gibbs slap," Cait confessed. The famous Gibbs on TV's *NCIS*, the number-two addiction Cait and I shared after Ben and Jerry's Heath Bar Crunch. The chief naval investigator played by Mark Harmon treats his motley fellow investigators with a mixture of impatience and candid affection. His trademark when they've done something stupid is the "Gibbs slap," a light whack to the back of their heads, which was what I had done in a frustrated moment.

"Would you mind explaining that to them when you go in tomorrow so they don't think I beat you?"

"Sure. I'm sorry."

"Yeah, right."

Cait sidled over to me and lowered her voice pretending to be Mark, "Do you want me to Gibbs slap you?" and then laughed. It was her standard joke whenever she was in a playful mood. This time I didn't laugh back.

The next day Cait met with her case manager to discuss her frustration over homework and the famous Gibbs slap that had me envisioning a call from child protection services. I couldn't help thinking about Meg Kelleher, Cait's kindergarten teacher, and the tap that led to her tearful confession. Now it was my turn. Being a good Catholic girl (up until I graduated parochial school at age twelve) I had carried around my guilt, complete with visions of fire and brimstone, for every sin. The effects of my Gibbs moment brought me back and led me to confess to anyone who'd listen and offer me absolution for my latest lapse in judgment. I had entered the "been there, done that crazy-mom zone." From that point forward, when my frustration level over homework was rising, I knew to leave the room and check back later, giving us both a chance to cool off.

The following Tuesday evening we settled in for an episode of *NCIS*. We laughed as character, Tony DiNozzo, said something we knew was going to get him in trouble with Gibbs and earn him a cuff to the back of his head.

"You gotta love Gibbs," chimed in Cait.

"Yup, ya sure do gotta love him."

16

OUT ON A LIMB

At Cait's small high school, the graduating class rarely topped seventy. It was hard not to know everyone. When Cait showed up for her first day of school, she was preceded by her IEP, the individual educational plan that specified her learning differences and stipulated modifications and accommodations for her. One of those accommodations was an educational assistant, who followed Cait through the day, explaining the many subtle and overt behaviors that even a twelve-page plan couldn't document.

Cait's eighth-grade English teacher was Mr. Caldwell. He was a pleasant enough man, though a little on the cool side. I noticed a slight edginess and a rigidity that made him hard to warm up to. He taught literature, theater, and writing: the last being Cait's nemesis. Whenever I encountered him at an open house or a meeting related to Cait's education plan, I felt a little intimidated by his demeanor. How would this cold fish connect with my daughter? Miraculously, Cait made it through all his assignments with help from her assistant and me until the day I got the call from Ann Wells, her case manager.

"Mr. Caldwell has some questions regarding Cait's most recent project."

Cait has just passed in an "All About Me" poster. "He's questioning the amount of help she received."

My face was burning. I wondered if she could feel its heat on the other end of the line. Didn't Mr. Caldwell read her IEP? I used my nicest, most persuading voice. "Ann, Cait possesses the fine motor and cutting skills of a kindergartener. This is high school. Do you think for a minute I'd allow her work to come in looking like the wall hanging of a snowflake cut out at preschool?" I refused to feel guilty about helping my daughter achieve a poster she could take pride in. I wasn't done. I laughed into the phone. "I'll help with her posters in college if I have to." Little did I know how often that would happen. I had no doubt Ann communicated my sentiments to Mr. Caldwell. He acquiesced and we moved on. It was a small victory after so many losing battles.

Cait managed to avoid Mr. Caldwell's classes again until she got into high school and needed an elective. Caldwell offered a theater class and since Cait's theatrics were pretty famous at home, she signed up. It helped that essays and posters weren't among the requirements.

The school had access to the town's Eclipse Grange, a nineteenth-century white, clapboard building, used by our town's theater troupe since the late 1960s. Its second story was chock full of costumes. I knew Cait would do cartwheels of joy once she got a glimpse of all the potential fantasy that lay in wait.

Any time I asked how class was going with Mr. Caldwell, Cait would give me a thumbs up. I was hopeful theater was going to be one less class for me to fret about. They did a lot of script reading in between theater exercises and games. It sounded like fun. I never remotely expected that my anxiety over Cait would play out in the reverse, and it would be Mr. Caldwell, not my daughter, I'd have to worry about. When I reflect back on the spring day that almost became Mr. Caldwell's unraveling, it seemed only natural that it would read back like a script written for its leading actress—Cait.

*   *   *

OUT ON A LIMB

CAST: Learning Specialist, Ann Wells
        Instructor, Dave Caldwell (Mr. C.)
        The Girl
        Student 1
        Student 2
        Four cast members

Act I, Scene 1

(High school corridor, early afternoon. Leaning against the doorframe of the cramped quarters of the special education office, MR. C. stands with shoulders slightly slumped. ANN WELLS looks up from her computer screen sensing trouble.)

ANN: Dave, come in. You look like you've had a rough day.

MR. C: *(lifting his hand, he rubs his forehead as though it has just started to throb)* In two decades of teaching, I thought I'd seen every thing.

ANN: *(gets up and pulls a chair out from the table)* Come sit.

MR. C: *(enters room and melts into the chair)* Look, I'm still shaking. *(holds up hand)*

ANN: *(looks at his outstretched fingers)* Jesus, Dave. What happened?

MR. C: I've just experienced one of the scariest moments of my entire teaching career. I feel like I've aged a lifetime.

ANN: *(hesitating)* Was it one of my students?

MR. C: *(looking right at her)* Who do you think?

Act II, Scene 1

(Earlier in the day, inside the grange. Mr. C. and several students gather in front of a small stage. In front of them, wooden seats are arranged in rows rising up to a platform where the stage lights are controlled. Several students are onstage rearranging the scenery.)

MR. C: Okay, listen up.

(Everyone stops what they are doing.)

MR. C: Amos and Colin, let's rehearse your scene next. The rest of you can take a quick stretch, but don't wander too far. The last scene includes everyone.

(Students scatter except for the two boys left on stage.)

Act II, Scene 2

(Outside the grange, a few minutes later. Several students are sitting on the steps. Two boys walk over to a large maple beyond the grange's porch. They are holding scripts. The Girl follows them. She has her script and a book. The boys sprawl out on the grass and talk about sports. The Girl stands on the other side of the tree and looks up.)

THE GIRL: *(announcing to no one in particular)* I'm going up.

(The two boys ignore her and remain immersed in their conversation.)

Act II, Scene 3

(Inside the grange, thirty minutes later. Students wander in. Mr. C. is up on the stage.)

MR. C: Gather round. *(scanning the group in front of him)* Who's missing?

(The cast looks at each other and shrug. Mr. C. shakes his head and turns toward the two students flanking his right—the same two boys who had been sitting under the tree earlier.)

MR. C: *(annoyed)* Go find her! I need you back here in two minutes. Hurry.

Act II, Scene 4
(Outside the grange. Student One and Student Two are standing on the porch looking out. Suddenly, they turn to each other and then back in the direction of the tree.)

STUDENT ONE: Who wants to tell Mr. C.?

STUDENT TWO: I'm not telling.

(They both hurry over to the tree.)

STUDENT ONE: Holy crap! You've got to get down!

THE GIRL: I can't!

(The grange door opens and MR. C., followed by several students, walks across to where the two boys are standing.)

MR. C: What on Earth—oh, for Christ sakes! What are you doing up there?

THE GIRL: I thought it was a good place to read.

(MR. C. stands directly under THE GIRL.)

MR. C: Get down right now.

THE GIRL: I'm stuck. I'm scared!

(An audible chuckle can be heard coming from the cast. MR. C. looks in their direction.)

CAST: *(silence)*

MR. C: *(removing a handkerchief from his back pocket, he wipes the sweat off his brow)* Hold on and steady yourself. Move one foot at a time. You can do it. I'm right here.

STUDENT ONE: Do you want me to get help?

(There's a slight rustling in the leaves.)

MR. C: *(looking up)* What are you doing!

(Opening his arms, he barely catches THE GIRL as she free falls past several limbs. He breaks her descent and staggers for a minute before he's able to lower her onto the ground.)

CAST: *(audible gasp)*

STUDENT TWO: Holy cow!

(Visibly shaken, MR. C. places his hands are on his hips and bends his head. After a minute, he lifts his head and turns towards THE GIRL.)

MR. C: Don't ever do anything like that again! You could have killed yourself!! *(turning to the rest of the cast)* Back inside. We've one more scene to rehearse.

Act III, Scene 1
(Inside the high school. Late afternoon in the learning center office.)

MR. C: She could have broken her damn neck.

ANN: What's that line actors use? Break a leg?

(For the first time that afternoon, MR. C. smiles.)

*　　　*　　　*

The evening of the show the small theater was packed with parents and students for the annual performance of short one-act plays. This year's was titled *Imperfect Pairs*. I couldn't help but think of Mr. Caldwell and my own daughter fitting the bill perfectly. Selfishly, from my end, if Cait had to experience a tree incident, I'm glad it was on his watch and not mine. I've no doubt he was far better at catching than me, and his anger regarding her actions that day would have a greater impact. Getting the call from Ann later that afternoon shook me, but I was grateful Mr. Caldwell didn't hold a grudge and let her continue with the play.

He had cast her perfectly. Her performance on stage required minimal memorizing, but offered an opportunity for Cait to become an otherworldly character, Galatea, the ivory statue that Pygmalion had carved and fallen in love with. In the Greek myth, Aphrodite, the goddess of love, takes pity on Pygmalion and brings the statue to life. Ethereal in her white toga and wreath of leaves and flowers, my very own Galatea certainly came to life. It was hard at times not to fall in love with her, even as she did mindless things and scared the crap out of us.

Opening night, I wondered if I should have sneaked a well-deserved bottle of wine to Mr. C., along with a short note— "Great catch!"

Cait would take a class with Mr. Caldwell again—senior English seminar. He would become one of her most valued teachers. She would learn to reflect on the written words before her, even her own. While there were teachers who still doubted Cait's analytical skills, Mr. Caldwell came to appreciate Cait, to see beyond her sometimes-outlandish behavior. One day in class, Cait got what no one else had picked up on. Later, Mr. Caldwell approached Ann, not as a man outdone, but as a proud teacher, sharing the triumph of his student.

In the end, I'd have to admit, he eventually caught on to Cait, and for that he got my rave review.

17

IT'S NOT ALWAYS ABOUT THE DRESS

Part of my together time with Cait was the drive to and from her school. One morning I spotted a sign alongside the school's entrance:

10th Grade
School Dance
Friday Night
7:30-11 p.m.

"Cait, check it out. There's a dance next Friday night." I was always on the lookout for social opportunities where I could plug her into a social event with her peers.

Silence.

I pushed a little further, "Want to go?"

"No."

Well, that was a dead end.

"Come on, Cait. It will be fun. Your sister used to love them." That was true, but I hated them when Courtney was in high school. By the time she could drive herself, she and her friends used dances as an excuse to meet up and take off for unchaperoned parties down the road.

Cait wasn't her sister. "I'm not going."

I learned early on there was little I could say or do when she had her mind made up. And her mind was made up in seventh grade: no dances. I knew the music was loud and for someone with sensory issues that meant deafening. I was well aware it wasn't any fun going to a dance alone. Yet, it never stopped me from asking each month when the sign appeared. I was more than a little surprised, therefore, when she got into the car one afternoon and announced, "There's a semiformal dance in March for juniors. I really want to go to it."

"Wow, Cait, that's great." I took my eyes off the road for a second to check out the girl sitting next to me. Is this Cait talking?

"I'll need a dress, you know, a long one," she gushed.

"We'll have to make a plan to go shopping for one."

"How about this weekend?"

The dance was a whole month away, but if all it took to get her to socialize was a dress, I was on it.

The following Saturday we began the search. She was adamant about what she didn't want, which was about every dress on the rack in the half dozen stores we went looking in. I knew Cait possessed an amazing imagination and undoubtedly had already visualized the perfect dress. I quickly realized our trip wasn't just about finding a dress; it was also about letting go of a dress that didn't exist.

A purple dress on the rack stood out. "Hey Cait, over here." It was her color, short skirt with spaghetti straps at the shoulders. Not even a smile from her direction.

"No way."

I went back to looking.

"Mom, over here!" I turned to see Cait holding up a killer gown: scarlet satin, long, and elegant. I peeked at the tag.

"This is way too expensive."

I didn't let on, that for a few seconds she and the dress tugged at my heartstrings. Still, I knew any formal gown had a life span of one night. I quickly turned and moved to the next rack ignoring her grumbling.

A store later she found it. I stared into the dressing room mirror watching her flirt back at her refection. Long, black, and strapless, it was layered with a shear material that shimmered like the night sky. It gave off a red carpet feel. It was still over budget, but Cait positively glowed. Sold.

Cait's luck with the dress didn't end there. Though Patrice, her Crafty Girls mentor, had moved to Cape Cod, her daughter, Emma, was returning for the dance. Once a classmate of Cait's, she offered to help get our Cinderella ready.

We picked up Emma at the bus station the afternoon of the dance. Back at the house, they immediately headed up the stairs. Occasionally, I'd hear giggles coming from Cait's room. The door was half open, but I knocked anyway. "Hey guys, can I come in?"

"Sure," they called out in unison.

Cait's room was anything but a typical teen's. It still looked like it did when she was ten. Cramped with stuffed animals, every other available space was occupied by Pokeman cards, fantasy books, and rock and shell collections. Her CD player, used only as a sleep aid to listen to storyteller Odds Bodkins, was now cranked up playing Alicia Keys, compliments of Emma.

The two girls had a mirror propped up against a chair and were kneeling down to apply mascara and lipstick while large curlers dangled from their heads.

"Pictures?" I wanted to record the moment.

Emma laughed, "Why not," and resumed applying her makeup while I took a few candid shots, proof that Cait had entered a new phase in adolescent life.

I left as quietly as I had entered, leaving them to their primping.

A half hour later they called out, "Here we come!"

Cait waltzed down the stairs, ahead of Emma, modeling her dress for me. She had the runway walk down, savoring each moment of her transformation. Emma knew the right amount of eye shadow and lipstick to define Cait's fine features. Her straight, dark blonde hair swept under her chin to frame her face. She had sneaked a red garnet necklace of her sister's. She was elegant.

I asked Cait what she'd wear over her dress. It was still March. She quickly retrieved a second hand, black leather jacket. It was the "old" Cait, but it added another dimension of cool to her outfit.

After a quick second photo shoot, we piled back into the car and were off to the gym.

"Emma. You're amazing. Thanks for this." She smiled and tucked her arm around Cait's.

It felt like only minutes since I had walked back in the house, kicked off my shoes and put up a pot for tea when the phone rang. "Come pick me up. I'm done."

"You just got there. Did you even dance?"

"Yes, with a bunch of kids, but I'm ready to come home." Her voice was firm. I knew there was no convincing her to stay longer.

As soon as I pulled into the parking lot, she was out the gym door and in the car. "How was it?"

"Great." She still had a can of open soda in her hand.

"Are you sure you want to leave?"

What the heck happened?

"I'm sure. I'm really tired."

Tired? Tired from what?

"Glad you went?"

I hope someone didn't say something stupid to her.

"Yessssss, I had fun."

Five minutes of fun. Well, I guess it trumps zero. I'll take it.

As we drove home she confined, "I felt pretty silly trying to dance in my dress. I couldn't move."

"Oh, no. Bummer."

"Yeah, I think I'm really a wallflower when it comes to dances."

I'm not sure what I was expecting. Her dress could have been entered into the *Guinness Book of World Records* under "Shortest Time Dress Worn at Semiformal High School Dance." But Cait went. How long she stayed didn't matter.

A month before Cait's graduation, there would be another dance and another dress. For her senior prom she even had a date—

Christian. Earlier in the year, she had met him at a teen gathering hosted by Vermont's Department of Disability, Aging, and Independent Living, which is open to high school students with all kinds of disabilities including Asperger's. The two hit it off and got together several more times during the year. As Cait's prom was approaching, I encouraged her to invite him.

After some cajoling she made the call. Christian was thrilled to be her escort. He hadn't gone to his own prom. His mom drove him the hour to our house, where Cait was waiting. His cerebral palsy showed in his awkward gait and halted speech, but in his suit and tie he appeared tall, dark, and handsome. His green eyes danced as he entered the house.

Cait's dress was new: still black, like the one before it, only this time, short and full, with room to dance. Her sister filled in for Emma, making sure she had the right color eye shadow and the mascara was applied without smudges. I charged the camera the night before, hoping to capture each moment of her debut. Cait's hair, now long, curled over her shoulders, framing long pearl earrings, which matched the white, satin sash of her dress. I became suddenly aware, for the first time, that her smile with Christian was flirtatious. When she posed with him, she held his arm, standing close.

Before leaving for the dance, Christian helped Cait put on a wrist corsage with a single white rose. She brought it slowly up to her nose, closed her eyes, and then without moving her hand, looked at him.

"Christian. It's beautiful. Thanks."

It was the stuff that dreams were made of—and mine, for that one instant, came true. My daughter was actually going to her prom, looking beautiful, with a lovely young man at her side.

I chauffeured them to the Davenport Inn. I debated driving home, remembering the semiformal dance, but decided to anyway.

It wasn't long after that the phone rang. I knew who was on the other end before I picked up. They had already eaten and danced—in record time—and were ready to be fetched. When I arrived in front of the building, they were waiting inside the doorway and walked out arm in arm. As I listened to their affectionate whispers in the backseat driving home, I knew what Cait now knew too. When a dance comes along, it's not always about the dress.

18

SISTER ACT

Cait's favorite class in high school was science. She'd cross the open courtyard, dash into the science lab, and be perched on her stool long before her fellow classmates entered. The buzz of their conversation when they arrived didn't interest her. Instead, her attention was on the windowsill lined with aquariums and cages that housed various critters. Cait had already taken several courses from Mr. Whitehall, the instructor. It was a small school. If you took more than one life science class, it usually meant having the same instructor again, or maybe even several times. Mr. Whitehall appreciated Cait's enthusiasm. In seventh grade, he allowed her to hatch baby chicks for her science project. He awarded her with the classroom key, so she could go in over the weekend to check on their progress. She won first place in the science fair that year.

On one particular day, a boy sitting at the table behind Cait noticed her talking to the small black and white bunny, Oreo.

When she came back over to sit down, he called out to her. "Hey, Cait."

She ignored him and pulled out her notebook. Mirroring her science partner, she opened it to yesterday's assignment, a strategy she learned to help keep her on track.

"Cait," he called again, "Today we're going to dissect a raaabiiit." He let the last word come out slowly. "My rabbit is going to be Oreo. I'm going to kill that bunny."

Cait swung around ready for battle. "You fucking go near the rabbit and I'll beat the shit out of you!"

"Oh, geez," Cait's lab partner mumbled and shook her head. Several other students nearby giggled.

Whitehall, who was passing out papers, came up the aisle and stopped. "What's going on here?"

Flushed, Cait clenched her fists, "He said he's going to kill Oreo!"

"I didn't say a word, Mr. W. Honest."

"He's lying!" The tears that had started to well up in her eyes spilled over.

I never knew all the details of the Oreo episode, but I had enough to let my imagination fill in the rest.

Several boys knew Cait was an easy target, especially when it came to animals. It was undoubtedly what led to the howling dogs that sometimes followed Cait as she walked to the library after school. Whitehall instinctively knew how to talk to Cait; he was a genuinely caring man. I wasn't sure if Mr. W. put an end to all the teasing in his class, but I was certain he championed Cait's side of the story that day.

In small New England towns, much of the local news can be learned in one of three places: the general store, the recycling center on Saturday mornings, or the hairdresser's.

I kept up with my news about every five weeks, when I had my hair foiled, colored, and cut. An entire head weighted down by sheaths of aluminum held me prisoner for an hour. There was no place to run or turn. I was forced to face my reflection while catching up on local gossip. My hairdresser's daughter was in Cait's class.

"How's Cait doing?"

"Okay. What about Krissy?"

"Same." After a telling hesitation, she continued. "Hey, I wanted you to know . . . Krissy said sometimes kids say mean things to Cait in bio class." She lifted her eyes to meet my own in the mirror.

"Really?"

She nodded and looked back down at my metallic head.

Sadly, the fun of teasing Cait followed her to biology. Everyone liked Mr. Sully. He was high energy, funny, and completely engrossed in his subject. He took his responsibility to impart knowledge seriously. This also made him a little less observant about what was going on under his radar, making it the perfect set up for picking on Cait.

I wanted to ask my hairdresser if Krissy did anything about it. Did she tell the teacher? Did she ask the kids causing the trouble to stop? I knew the answer. Krissy was painfully shy. She would have a hard time calling attention to herself, or worse, she would inadvertently redirect the teasing her way. I didn't wait for my hairdresser's answer. "Thanks for telling me, and please thank Krissy. It helps to know what's going on."

Without names or details, there wasn't much I could do. When I approached Cait with it, she shrugged me off. Perhaps she was oblivious to the more subtle comments made behind her back. I wanted to help my daughter, but I didn't want to be *that* parent. I was an educator and well aware of staff reaction. "Oh no, *she's* here . . . again." But maybe, I had it all wrong. I didn't have to wait long to find out.

On Tuesday Cait had a meltdown in bio. "You are such jerks!" There was no mistaking the origin of the accusation.

Across the table from Cait were two boys. "Dave, look! Is this a pathetic looking specimen or what?" He flipped the earthworm, which was today's lab, over to his friend.

"Let's chop it up in a million pieces and serve it for lunch."

By now, Cait was standing. She reached across and grabbed the first thing she could, Dave's notebook, and flung it across the aisle. She was out the door before Dave or his friend even had a chance to blink.

Unlike her previous teacher, Mr. Sully immediately called for Cait's assistant, who in an effort to foster greater independence, wasn't in class with her. Together they quickly made the decision for Cait to remain outside the class, with Mr. Sully, while her assistant explained to her classmates why Cait had gotten upset. When I found out, Cait's anger quickly transferred over to my own. I was outraged. All my old feelings of having her become "the hallway kid" flooded back.

Then and there I vowed that it was the last time Cait would be singled out. Now, she wasn't only the brunt of a schoolboy's joke. She had been held outside the room, setting her even further apart. And by discussing her behaviors with the class, her assistant bordered a breech in confidentiality. Though I knew she had the best intentions, and her loyalties lied with Cait, she had shared things about Cait behind her back. I hated it as much as I hated the teasing. I knew both her teacher and assistant were acting in what they thought was Cait's best interest, but it felt wrong.

Somewhere in the midst of my frustration over what had happened, I began to rally around the idea of educating Cait's classmates about Asperger's, hoping it would help to empower my daughter. I didn't have a clue, though, as to how I was going to do it. I knew I needed to find the right person to help me. Since I was just another annoying parent, and Cait's assistant was seen as her school bodyguard, I had to think outside the box. I realized pretty quickly Courtney was the best shot at creating a bridge of understanding between Cait and her peers.

The idea of asking her big sister for help took root after watching the movie *Intricate Minds,* which was a story, told by kids, about kids with Asperger's. Courtney was currently between jobs. The timing was perfect. While home one day, I put the question to her.

"Hey, how would you like to help explain your sister's Asperger's?"

She looked at me like I had lost it. "Explain her Asperger's? And to whom pray tell?"

"Her classmates."

"How exactly are you thinking I should do that?"

I made her watch the film with me that night.

"God, this is so cheesy." She complained, but she didn't flatly refuse—a good sign.

Though Courtney and Cait's relationship had always been close, like many siblings it was peppered with moments of frustration and disapproval. Their age difference provided enough of a buffer that at least Courtney's friends saw Cait as cute and quirky, but in Courtney's eyes Cait's behavior was not always quite so benign.

"Cait, look. Jay bought you a gift for Christmas." Courtney's current boyfriend had included her sister in his gift giving.

As Cait unwrapped the parcel she let loose an audible sigh, "I don't particularly like this movie." Her sister, using Herculean constraint to stop herself from lurching across the living room to strangle Cait, wouldn't speak to her for the rest of the day. Jay, on the other hand, laughed it off and ended up exchanging it for a book she wanted instead. From that point forward, Cait had to rehearse with her sister any and all boyfriend encounters until Courtney was satisfied. Still, when Cait entered a room and Court's boyfriend was there, we all held our breath.

Though my oldest born never admitted it, I knew there were times she longed for a sister who she could cheer for at sporting events, advise on clothes or share secrets about boys and dating with. I also recognized that Courtney was smart enough to make her peace early on, and she learned that humor and a short memory could get her through some of the more dicey "Cait" moments. Despite sisterhood challenges, their bond and loyalty grew. It was an odd relationship. Courtney was the consummate seeker of social approval and sensed the nuances of a situation from a mile away. Cait was clueless that the world outside her head didn't read her mind, and she certainly had no desire to read anyone else's.

When I approached Cait's school team about having her sister come in to lead a discussion on Cait's challenges, surprisingly, they supported it and helped put things in motion.

The day the two sisters went to school together, Cait was all nerves, while Courtney was calm and confident. She possessed a respectable past at her alma mater: good student, formidable athlete, popular with teachers and peers—many of whose younger siblings would now be sitting in front of her. As my two daughters drove off that day, I couldn't help thinking this could be Cait's first day of acceptance and belonging. I silently prayed I had made the right choice.

When I arrived home from work later that afternoon, I flew from the driveway into our house. "Tell me! Tell me everything! Did it go okay? Don't leave out any details."

I found them both curled up together on the couch watching a DVD, "Shhhh, this is the good part." Cait was in her "can't you see I'm in the middle of a movie" zone. I wouldn't get any information out of her.

Instead, I whispered over her head, "Court, into the kitchen."

I must have looked desperate. Without the need for a second plea, Courtney got off the couch and followed me.

"I'm dying to hear. How did it go?"

"Good."

"Good? Come on, Court. I've been a wreck all day."

"Okay, okay." She poured herself a glass of lemonade. I would have poured myself a glass of wine, but it was four in the afternoon.

"I thought it went really well," emphasizing the "r" in "really." "We started in creative writing. I asked the class what came to mind when they thought of someone with a learning challenge. They talked about struggling with reading and writing reports. Then there's this guy in the back who shouts out that he stinks at math."

"So does half the population." I couldn't resist the punch line.

Courtney gave me her "who's telling this" look. "It was a good icebreaker because they all started to laugh. We talked about how physical challenges are a lot easier to recognize, like someone in a wheelchair, or with a service dog. Everyone admitted it was easier to be tolerant of someone with a physical handicap than it was to accept someone who was socially challenged. And that's when we opened it up to Cait."

She stopped to sip of her lemonade, "You know mom, they're not stupid. They knew where this was heading, so I moved quickly, I didn't want to lose them. I said we were there to talk about some of Cait's challenges, which they might have noticed, but maybe found confusing. We watched a few minutes of the film and talked about how having Asperger's is not unlike being dyslexic. Instead of learning to read the words on a page, Cait is learning to read social situations and check her responses. And just like you don't outgrow being dyslexic, you don't outgrow Asperger's, but you can learn to cope."

Courtney opened the fridge to scope out last night's leftovers. I worked hard to be patient. As she closed the door, she laughed. "When I asked Cait if she liked dances . . ."

Just then her sister walked into the kitchen and belted out a resounding, "NO!"

Courtney shot her a look, "That got a good laugh from the class!"

Cait sat on a kitchen stool to make her presence known, but she let Courtney continue. "Crowded places and sometimes even the hallways bother you, right Cait? We said that if they magnified the noise level ten times, that's what Cait hears."

"And there you have it," mimicked Cait in her announcer's voice.

"So, we just talked about the stuff that Cait finds difficult, you know . . ." Courtney turned to Cait and lowered her voice, "like picking her skin in class when she's anxious."

Cait ignored this. "Tell her about getting ready for a date."

Courtney rolled her eyes for my benefit. "I told them that though I love my sister, she makes me crazy. She never holds back what she's thinking and is always honest, well honest most of the time." Courtney knew all about Cait's thievery impulses and trip to the police station. "Yes, Cait can get herself in hot water with me."

Cait didn't miss her cue and repeated what she said in class, "Well, don't you want me to tell you that your dress doesn't look good?"

"Not really, Cait." Courtney turned to me, "That got another good laugh."

"But Cait," she looked back at her sister, "We also talked about your loyalty, and that you don't talk behind people's backs." Courtney paused, then continued, "We said Asperger's isn't an excuse to be rude, Cait, and if you say something hurtful, your classmates should tell you, but in a respectful way."

"Agreed," chimed Cait.

"And, Cait, they now know that you believe what people tell you. You have a hard time understanding sarcasm."

"Yeah, like Pete saying he was going to kill Oreo."

"It was great Pete was there to hear that. I think we nailed him on that one."

Cait laughed.

Courtney shared that when it was the class's turn to ask questions, one boy asked why Cait never told them she had Asperger's. Someone else told Cait she never knew either.

"And . . ." I needed to know how it ended.

"Nobody wants to go around with a label, but we explained it was why we were there to discuss it today. Right, Cait?"

Cait stood up. "Right."

Courtney added, for my benefit, "I thought it went really well. So did her teachers, and a few kids even thanked us."

As the two sisters stood side-by-side, with the late afternoon light streaming into the kitchen, Cait put her arms around her sister, "You're the best, Court."

Courtney hugged her back, "I'd say we make a pretty darn good team."

19

THE ADVOCATE

I was beginning to feel like I had grown a new appendage—the telephone. As soon as I got home from school each day, I would park myself next to it and work my way down an ever-changing list of numbers. It felt like I had spoken to every available resource person in the state. The conversation would always start in the same way. "Hi, I was wondering if you could help me. I'm the parent of an Asperger's student attending high school and need some guidance."

Sometimes the person I was calling would immediately redirect me, while other times they'd listen with a sympathetic ear, leaving me no further ahead, but feeling temporarily better. I spoke to one parent group run by professionals in Burlington, Vermont. They offered evening workshops, which were too far away for me to attend. After scribbling out the various helpful suggestions and hanging up, I still felt ill equipped to act on them. Some of those afternoon calls led me to the state's Department of Education where I quickly discovered that they worked through the school's administration, a department I no longer trusted.

The list finally led me to Sonya, a special education advocate. She had helped an acquaintance of mine in a neighboring district, whose daughter had a complex profile with multiple needs. My case was simple by comparison. I wasn't looking for a fancy private school. Cait's three-year evaluation was coming up, which meant retesting. This would determine if she was still eligible for special education services. I was hoping for some good, solid recommendations that her school could follow—and that would mean involving experienced professionals. Though Cait wasn't overly complicated by some standards, her disability, Asperger's, was like the new kid on the block. My history so far at Cait's high school taught me one important thing: Good intentions didn't always equal good results.

Sonya set up a time and place for us to meet. She would be passing near where I lived, after visiting another client in the southern part of the state. She suggested the McDonald's just off the highway. When I entered the restaurant, I wasn't exactly sure what my new savior looked like. Luckily it was midafternoon and the lunch crowd had thinned out. I spotted a woman, with long dark hair, seated at a table next to the window. She was casually dressed and appeared to be in her late thirties, but the tip-off was the pile of folders next to her salad. "Sonya?"

"You must be Lyn." She smiled and motioned for me to join her. "If you don't mind, I'm only just now getting to my lunch."

"I'm glad you could fit me into your schedule." I glanced at the pile. "I see you got the paperwork I sent. Did you have a chance to go through it?"

I was anxious to get started and hoped she was willing to work between swallows. Her lunch was costing me. It was the most money I'd ever spent at McDonald's—fifty dollars an hour to be exact.

I had sent her all of Cait's previous reports and her current plan for services. I was frustrated and tired. I needed help.

"I looked through them. Why don't you start by telling me what's happening in Cait's program right now."

That would be easy. Not a lot.

I never thought I'd need to hire an advocate, but I was acutely aware of Cait's ticking clock. I wanted her to graduate prepared and ready for the next step, which I was hoping included college and friendship. "Sonya, do you think you can help us?"

"Absolutely. The next step is to let the team know I'll be present at your next meeting." With that she whipped out her calendar. Inwardly, I let out a deep exhale. I was running out of options, but now I finally had someone onboard who might make a difference.

As we walked out to the parking lot, I watched her get into an old Toyota Corolla wagon with rust starting to show. I knew she wasn't making millions at what she did, but as a single parent, I would be taking a financial hit with this change in tactics. As I drove off a few seconds later, I felt empowered for the first time, until images of my next high school meeting moved in and that old feeling of self-doubt took its place.

Instead of calling, I decided to email Ann Wells, Cait's case manager at school, and let her know that an advocate would be attending our next meeting. On the afternoon of the meeting, I met Sonya in the school's parking lot. We entered the building just as Ann was walking down the hall. I called her over to make introductions. She politely nodded, "The room is still in use. It will be a few more minutes." With that she kept walking.

Sonya and I glanced at each other. "I guess that was a little on the chilly side," I said apologetically.

"Don't worry, I'm used to it."

I wasn't. I knew having an advocate would change the tenor of our meetings, but it still caught me by surprise. I liked Ann. Normally she would talk up a storm, mostly about how busy and overworked she was. She had a big heart and cared about her charges, but Cait's needs were complicated. I hated ruffling Ann's or anyone's feathers. Even though parenting Cait required a whole new skill set, I was never comfortable when I was forced to use it. I guess that's why I decided to pay Sonya the big bucks.

When we finally gathered around the table, we were back in familiar territory, discussing math. Little had changed in Cait's math program since Aubrey Banks's reign as LEA. Her replacement was the assistant to the special ed director for the district. She seemed highly efficient and fair-minded. Time would tell.

Sonya placed a small tape recorder in the center of the table. "I hope everyone is okay with this."

Oh boy, this is going to go over big. Imagine if I had a recorder running during Aubrey's meetings! I could have saved some of her pearls for eternity.

"I find it helpful since sometimes things are missed when taking notes," Sonya reassured the group.

Notes? Should there have been notes from our previous meetings? I wondered if Ann ever wrote any up, especially when Sonya asked her if she might provide them from the last several times we had met. "Of course," Ann agreed without ever looking in her direction.

Sonya said little. My guess was that it was an advocate thing, like being a silent partner. The running tape recorder and her note taking, however, propelled us forward. She finally spoke, "I know this past fall Cait had achievement testing done outside the district. It appeared to have confirmed that her math reasoning and writing skills are weak."

Ann and the team acknowledged the testing I had spent my grocery money on. It was done by a highly reputable learning center in the area. The team then shared several math options and there was even discussion about attending another local high school math class where block scheduling was not an issue. I hoped as Sonya listened she would understand that, like so many suggestions, these sounded good, but probably wouldn't work. Sonya knew my biggest worry, I didn't want Cait's educational assistant, with no math background, tutoring her. At this point though, we were moving forward, albeit a few baby steps at a time.

The stakes would be higher at our next team meeting when we planned her three-year evaluation. The goal at a pre-evaluation is to propose questions that, when answered, will determine eligibility. The most important piece in determining Cait's eligibility would be the assessments used and the people administering them. We left agreeing on a day and time. Sonya was turning out to be an invaluable team member. Then I got her bill.

Maybe it wasn't large by others' standards, but it was to me. I immediately dialed her number. "Hi Sonya, I just wanted to confirm our next meeting time." Not wanting to alienate my ally, I decided not to start the conversation with "Five hundred dollars! *Seriously?*"

"I'm so glad you called. I think I might have a conflict, but I'm feeling at this meeting you'll be fine without me."

Are you joking? Why the hell do you think I've hired you?

"Actually, Sonya, this meeting is extremely important and I'll need you there to back me up. There are some key people I'd like to have test Cait." It appeared the issue was an earlier meeting in her schedule. I promised I'd contact the team and move ours back an hour.

"By the way, I just received your bill. Would you mind explaining it to me while I have you on the phone?" I used the cheeriest voice I could muster. It appears that I wasn't only paying for her enjoyment of a Mickey D salad, but also all phone calls, whether dialed or answered, email responses, and report readings, and finally time spent listening to iTunes as she drove between her house in central Vermont and our town eighty miles away. What I was thinking was static on the line was the "cha-ching" on her pocket calculator.

I was already in too deep to bail. I bit the bullet, "So, I'll see you Thursday, then," operating my own calculator to the tune of two hundred dollars for Thursday's meeting.

I didn't resent Sonya. I admired her. She found a niche and filled it. I should have realized all this during our initial conversation when she dropped lots of new educational buzzwords. She had gotten into advocating after her divorce when she found herself navigating the special education system alone for one of her own children. She contacted a friend who was familiar with special education law and quickly became self-taught in the twists and turns of student rights and services. Now she aided people like me, often getting them the help they needed.

But what was it that Cait needed exactly? This was the question I was constantly trying to get answered. Her high school wasn't a bad place. People were honest and worked hard. I believed they recognized Cait's unique profile and that she didn't fit into their usual package of services. As her mom, and greatest advocate, I didn't want them to simply push her through because they didn't know what else to do with her.

When Thursday finally rolled around, I was ready. I waited in the parking lot for Sonya. Please don't be late. When her beat-up Toyota rolled in, I took a deep breath. Together, once again, we headed into the building and the table that awaited us.

Sonya was familiar with the professionals in our area. We had agreed on the ones we felt were the most knowledgeable for testing Cait. "Listen, the best approach is to get them to come up with these people themselves."

"Oh, that will be easy," I murmured back with a touch of sarcasm.

What I liked about our new LEA was that she had the dual role of assistant director of special education. She listened. I didn't believe she was a push over, but she was smart. Just maybe she'll get it.

Sonya was right. We dropped a couple of names they knew and approved of, but there was hesitation with the speech and language pathologist. "Every district employs one, so why go outside?" the LEA pointed out.

I broke Sonya's rule and made my pitch. "There is one that has been recently trained in a social thinking program developed in California. It's very innovative and she's using it in her school district with great results." It was Kathryn who had come up with the concept of Crafty Girls.

"I've heard of it," the assistant director shared, confirming my first impression. "She would be able to test Cait and provide concrete recommendations based on a program that can help set measurable goals."

There was a quick exchange of smiles. All administrators loved words like measure and assess. I had to keep myself from breaking into a grin. I got us a crackerjack speech pathologist. But the real jackpot came when the assistant director turned to me, "It looks like you already had the achievement testing completed. The district will reimburse you the costs for that." I worked hard not leap up on top of the table and start dancing.

We agreed to have another meeting after all the testing was completed in order to determine eligibility and decide on Cait's program for her remaining couple of years of high school.

I walked Sonya to her car, "Thanks so much. It was a good meeting. Hopefully things will start to move forward."

"I think we've got ourselves a good team for Cait's evaluation. Keep me posted. I'll see you in a month or so."

I knew that I was parting company with Sonya in the parking lot that day. Her presence had communicated to the team that I was serious. Yet, I wondered if a six-foot, buff, male boxer would have done the same and cost less. I appreciated her efforts and I learned a few things, but at that point I knew I could continue the good fight on my own. After I paid my last bill, I called to thank her and wish her good luck.

The professionals who tested Cait did their job well, just as Sonya and I believed they would, and the team accepted and acted on their recommendations. Math was never fully resolved, but the district did pay for outside tutoring. In her senior year, Cait would take a class with a great teacher who helped her pass the math competencies required for graduation. The real coup was the team agreed Cait should join a group outside school for social thinking taught by the speech pathologist, who had tested her. The district agreed to pay for this, including sessions that were held during the summer months.

Unlike Arthur's Camelot, Cait and I couldn't conclude our story here with a happy ending. The journey continued along with more grumblings among Cait's knights who still struggled with their loyalties.

20

MORE THAN THE SUM OF MY PARTS

"Come on, Cait, you don't want to be late," I yelled back into the house. The snow was falling gently now, with a good six inches from the previous night already on the ground. I had just finished brushing the snow off the windows of my now heating car, hoping by the time we set out, the temperature would be above freezing. I didn't expect the town's snowplow had been down our road yet. It was Saturday—no school, which meant their usual 6:30 a.m. sweep would be more like nine o'clock instead. We needed to be at our destination by eight.

"I'm coming, I'm coming," came the irritable reply.

It was seven miles to the museum. I knew the turns and icy patches, where to slow down and shift into second, but the drive would not be easy. It was Cait's second year at the science museum, and we'd fallen into a weekend rhythm. It might have been nice to sleep-in occasionally on a Saturday, but that wasn't part of the plan. I debated where to go after dropping her off for my hour and a half wait until her shift ended. On a nicer morning there would have been more choices.

By the time we reached the end of our driveway Cait's mood lifted from sleepy and ill-tempered to awake and upbeat.

Sometimes we arrived before Loren, the museum's caretaker, and had to wait. Today, open gates greeted us. Good. I stopped the car in front of the entrance, twenty yards from the front door and waited to see if he'd remembered to unlock it. He had. Cait turned to wave as she slipped inside.

Ever since Cait had entered high school I had looked for ways to bring her out into the world. The local science museum seemed a perfect choice. She spent hours there when she was younger. A year ago she had begun as a volunteer. This new step had been a process, like everything else. First, I found Sarah, a local college big sister. College students were always looking for ways to bump up their community service hours. Jane, Cait's therapist, and an instructor at the school, made the connection for us. Sarah was lovely, and got along well with Cait. Having Jane on board made it seamless. She was able to field any questions Sarah had about Cait's disability.

For six months, Cait and I picked Sarah up outside her dorm room and then I would drop the two of them off at the museum. Sarah helped Cait figure out the jobs Loren set before them each week. Sometimes it was cleaning fresh water tanks, while other times it was reorganizing exhibits before the doors opened at 10:00 a.m. When the semester ended and Sarah could no longer fit Saturday mornings into her schedule, Loren took over. By then, Cait knew him well.

When I came back to pick her up that snowy day, I found the two of them outside shoveling the sidewalks together. Her cheeks were red, her eyes bright.

"Hey, how was it today?" I asked.

"Great, the fish nibbled at my fingers. It feels so cool when they do that."

"What else did you do?"

"I cleaned the ball machine. It was fun."

I couldn't imagine that cleaning steel balls was much fun, but Cait loved it. It was a huge Rube Goldberg contraption with a series of ramps and wheels. It fascinated Cait. Loren had to use a drill to remove the heavy plexiglass panels so that Cait could get at the twenty-five golf-sized balls and individually clean each one. Cait's biggest thrill was using the drill herself with Loren guiding the pieces as they came off.

I knew her two hours there every Saturday gave her a chance to be a little kid. She'd crawl through tunnels of the children's play center collecting misplaced toys or reorganizing the shelves of small plastic animals in the gift shop. Her favorite time was when Loren had her vacuum the exhibit shop rooms with a pack-like suction machine she carried on her back. I appreciated Loren's easy going way with her. Once when I picked her up, he called me over to come sit with him.

"Cait seemed a little uptight today. You know, she struggles to express what's troubling her. Is she seeing someone to talk through stuff that's bothering her?" He was always alert to Cait's moods as well as her interests. I assured him she had someone.

Cait had found her volunteer niche at school as well. It started out with her looking for a quiet place to have lunch. The cafeteria was tiny and a lot of students ended up eating along the corridor. It was too busy for Cait. Nearby was a classroom for two special need students, Annabel and Tamara. Somehow, Cait found her way into their space and made it her daily ritual to eat with them. Their teachers welcomed her, as she seemed to have a special connection with their two charges. Neither girl could speak. Annabel signed. Tamara had a voice recorder.

"You should have seen how excited Annabel was today," Cait shared one afternoon.

"What were you guys doing?"

"I brought in a butterfly for her to look at. It landed on her arm. She loved it!"

One day I asked, "Cait, why do you like being with Tamara and Annabel so much?"

"They're like me—different."

My heart broke. These girls were remarkably dissimilar from one another, and unlike Cait, too. Yet, this was how she saw herself in comparison to everyone else.

At the same time I was fiercely proud of her. It was at these moments that Cait was the model child—completely devoid of judgment, never setting herself apart or above somebody else. Her time with Annabel and Tamara during lunch gave her as much as she gave back. Cait liked these girls and didn't feel sorry for them, any more than she did for herself. She didn't see that having lunch with them was volunteering. Maybe she enjoyed Annabel and Tamara because, like her, they didn't judge.

At the end of each year, when awards were given out, Cait always earned one for her volunteer work. It was the only time she stepped up to the podium.

While other high school students had after-school or weekend jobs, I knew that wasn't going to happen with Cait. There weren't a lot of Sarahs walking around who could teach her the ropes, or employers like Loren, willing to take the time. But, one day, amazingly, she did find work.

Cait happened to be in the school office when Elsa walked in. Elsa, who lived in town and had a son at Cait's school, had just posted a "Help Wanted" sign. She was looking for someone to help her with her fledgling pet-sitting business. Cait saw the sign and quickly ran out of the building, chasing after Elsa.

"Wait up!" she hollered. By the time Cait caught up to Elsa, her excitement was over the top. "I'm interested! I love animals, all kinds. I always wanted to babysit, for animals that is."

"Go home and ask your mom. Then call me. We'll talk more." And with that she drove off.

The next afternoon, Cait had me on the phone arranging a time to go over to Elsa's for an interview.

I gave it to Cait straight, "Tell Elsa about your Asperger's. It's important for her to know."

When we arrived, there was no need to ring the doorbell. Three dogs came bounding to the screen door, barking loudly, followed by Elsa, who was calmly quieting them down. She led us into her living room. I don't think there was a square inch that wasn't covered in dog hair. I sat on the edge of her couch while Cait plopped right down in the middle and immediately began to say hello to every furry creature that greeted her. The house was disheveled, a little like Elsa, herself, but Elsa's love for her dogs was apparent. Cait shared a little bit about her challenges and Elsa asked good questions.

"How is having Asperger's a challenge for you?"

"Paying attention is hard, and sometimes being around people when they're all talking at once."

"Is that why you love animals so much?"

"Yes," replied Cait looking down at the cat snuggled in her lap. "Have you ever read the book *All Cats Have Asperger's*?" Cait asked.

"No, tell me about it." After listening, Elsa shared that she thought her son had some similar issues. She hired Cait on the spot.

Cait established her new routine and took the school bus to Elsa's two afternoons a week. She was ecstatic. It wasn't about having a job, or even receiving a paycheck. It was spending time with Elsa and her menagerie of critters that made her glow.

When I'd pick her up, she would be excited about what she'd done that day. Elsa's newly rescued golden retriever, Echo, was in training for future use as a therapy dog. Cait would accompany Elsa to training classes and at other times help her with the pet-care service. Their relationship lasted over a year, until Elsa moved away.

Cait was starting to let others in and beginning to reach out. All these people touched her life in ways I couldn't. I was grateful and surprised that they not only understood my daughter, but also appreciated her differences. I wanted to remember them and I wanted Cait to remember them too: Sarah, her college big sister, who willingly rose early every Saturday to accompany her to the museum; Loren and the prized "ball machine;" Tamara and Annabel with their smiles; and Elsa's precious Echo. How much fun it would be to wear their special charms on a bracelet, to listen to them jingle, to watch their reflection dance in the light. There were many more charms that would follow, but the most amazing charm of all was Cait herself.

21

BUSTED

There was not one person in Cait's school career, except for Aubrey Banks, the infamous Morgan le Fay, whom I did not respect, nor believe had Cait's best interests at heart. They simply didn't have experience working with someone with Asperger's. Since parenting a child with Asperger's was new to me as well, I couldn't fault them for that, but I did have one gripe; they never considered using a trained specialist to directly support Cait's academics. I believed she needed a qualified person to teach concrete strategies when approaching new writing and reading assignments. Her school said they were doing that by providing her with an educational assistant. It wasn't the same. We never saw eye-to-eye on this issue during her middle and high school years. At home, I picked up the slack and helped her play catch up, and on occasion, it got me into trouble.

My involvement in Cait's academics reached a crisis stage when she signed up senior year for a class on social issues with a focus on sustainability and food. I'm sure Cait thought what could be more fun than eating and taking another class with dreamy teacher, Kip. He was young with schoolboy charm and big blue eyes.

Cait first encountered Kip in her eighth-grade geography class. That was when her assistant was Tate, fresh out of AmeriCorps and fully committed to Cait's academic success. If Kip had any confusion over how to handle my daughter, Tate was on it.

By the time Cait was a senior, Tate was gone and her assistant no longer accompanied her to class. I wondered how she'd fair now.

"You're not going to believe what I saw today?" She had barely opened the car door.

"What?" A bird on her class window ledge?

"Do you know that people who work in slaughterhouses lose things? Things like limbs?"

"Ugh, that's awful."

"That's not all of it." She went on to paint me more grim images of Nebraska meatpacking plants. The readings and movies they watched in Kip's class portrayed graphic and upsetting realities, but to Cait these injustices were especially difficult. She didn't allow me to cook red meat for weeks.

I quickly caught on to the course's content and focus. This class was less about local cuisines and more about having students use their critical thinking skills to examine society's relationship with the food industry. It was my first red flag. I knew this would expose Cait's challenges as a linear thinker. It was a small class with a lot of discussion. It required thinking on your feet, not something Cait managed easily. To top it off, Kip liked to talk—a lot. In her struggle to stay focused, Cait used some less than desirable behaviors, the worst of them picking her skin. Jane, her therapist, explained it as a way Cait attempted to stay with it, like pinching herself awake. Cait would think nothing of pulling up the leg of her pants to pick away at the skin on her knee. It was a distraction, not to mention gross.

With graduation around the corner, Cait needed to pass Kip's class. I ordered one of the books Kip required them to read. I figured if she owned a copy she could write and highlight in it. I had us both reading it. Cait actually sponged the information, as if she were watching a sci-fi channel, but writing about the topics was altogether different. Kip piled on the assignments, making evenings when Cait had a Kip assignment, exhausting.

The next red flag came when her learning specialist called wanting to meet and asked that Cait be there, too. It wasn't unusual to have a check-in meeting, so I wasn't suspicious until I entered the crowded room where all her teachers for the semester had congregated, including the dean, who was leaning against a desk along the wall. I always insisted on Jane, her therapist's, presence with good reason. She was tuned into Cait, and could explain her behaviors to others. Cait sat between the two of us. I could feel Cait's anxiety rising with my own. Now what?

The dean, Mr. Miller, spoke up first. "Cait, I'm glad you could join us. I know it probably feels a little overwhelming. But you know all these people, so don't feel nervous." He's kidding, right?

The new learning specialist, Shelly Watts, had joined the dean. "Why don't we start by checking in and see how things are going for you this term. Let's hear from you first."

I had met with Shelly that summer to introduce myself and to share my wish list: work with my daughter on writing. It didn't happen. I was looking back and forth between this new tag team, Shelly and the dean, trying to decide whom I liked the least at this very moment.

One by one Cait's team members spoke their piece.

"Cait's doing well in English. She hasn't fallen behind on any assignments." Thank you, Mr. C.

It was Mr. Stevens's turn. "Cait occasionally gets distracted by some of the other students in my class who are chatty, but she's getting her work done." He shifted his gaze to the student sitting stone still next to me, "Nice job, Cait." You could always depend on Mr. Stevens to be honest.

"How are things going in your class, Kip?" Shelly interjected. I had enough intuition to figure we were finally getting to the real reason we were all here.

Kip hesitated. Oh for God sakes, just spill it. It finally dawned on me why I had a hard time connecting with Kip. It wasn't just that I had long ago outgrown my own school-girl crushes. Kip was a little like Cait. He was his own linear thinker. He lacked a ready sense of humor and the parenting perspective of teachers like Mr. C., who could save girls falling out of trees. I wondered if Kip would ever catch on to my daughter.

"Cait is really struggling with paying attention. It's a discussion class and Cait's behavior can be disruptive." He twisted around in his chair to face me. "Cait came in upset the other day. When I asked her about the homework assignment, she complained that she had been up very late, and shared that you ended up writing most of it." Busted.

I heard Jane shift in her chair. I felt both embarrassed and annoyed, but my annoyance won out. I turned to my daughter. "I know you're working hard, Cait, but it's important you work hard at paying attention, too. It's a long class. If you need to get up and move, ask permission to leave for a minute, but you need to try harder." It was the same old ninety-minute block dilemma, but I didn't want them to think I was letting Cait off the hook.

I swung back to Kip. "In Cait's afterschool social thinking program (which everyone here knows about, right?) there are tools to help with expected behaviors, like behavior mapping." I didn't tell him that the school was paying for this with the intention that Cait would use what she'd learned in her classes, including his.

I turned to Shelly, "The maps, done with a student, literally map out what a student hopes to achieve and where an unexpected versus expected behavior will land them. It's concrete. It teaches what most students intuitively pick up, but others don't." (like those with Apserger's!) I knew these were bright and caring adults, but in their presence I felt like I had just gotten caught with my hand in the cookie jar. It was one step away from a reprimand. "Cait and I will do one tonight for your class, Kip, and send it in tomorrow. Okay, Cait?"

She nodded.

I knew by now Cait had mentally checked out and was probably fantasizing about becoming a Ninja turtle. I wanted to join her, since I was pretty sure they weren't through with me yet.

We were back to Mr. Miller. "Lyn, we've some concern that Cait is feeling a lot of pressure from home and that you may be helping her too much."

Were we talking too much help from me or not enough help from school? I'm filling in the gaps! I thought, trying telepathically to reach Jane. I'm right, right? But she was looking at me waiting for the answer too.

I started to fantasize about what I really wanted to say. "Well, Mr. Miller, it's like this. Cait's trying the only way she knows how, but that's not going to make the grade as you well know. I mean seriously, Mr. Miller, what's a mother to do? Every night I have to crack the old whip and say, 'Get to it, Cait,' and not let up until the clock strikes midnight. Oh, and yes, there are times I just sit down in a heap of frustration and do that damn paper myself!"

But unlike Cait I had long ago passed Social Thinking 101. I understood only too well the intricacies of the situation we were now in.

"Mr. Miller, it is difficult in the evening." Play the victim, that usually works, I said to myself. "As I'm sure you know, Cait's meds have long since worn off and she's pretty spent." I glanced around at her teachers. "And yes, sometimes it's a struggle to get her to finish her work."

I looked in Cait's direction, but she was staring straight ahead having her own solitary monologue. I continued. "I don't really do her work." Bless me father for I have sinned. "I type for her and help her brainstorm." Lame. Cait nodded her agreement. So, why didn't she tell them that instead of' "my mom wrote it?"

Jane cleared her throat for attention. Finally.

"We know there are concerns about Cait managing her work load with the least amount of stress. Lyn is trying to compensate in areas that are especially challenging."

As I listened to Jane, I started to wonder why we were all actually there. What did this team really want? If it was to call me out on supporting Cait, what was the alternative?

Bless Jane. They all seemed to be listening. "I think everyone at this table understands, including you too, Cait, that moving up through the grades means greater demands, which may lead you to feel more anxious." Jane locked eyes with everyone on the team. "When you couple anxiety and attention challenges, the working memory is less able to help you think through a problem. Using the social mapping should help with this."

She swung back to Cait, "You know some stress is actually good, Cait. Without a little tension we'd never move to the next level. You've got a lot of caring adults who are here to support you in doing that." For once, the team agreed.

Cait and I went home that afternoon and mapped out behavior goals to assure greater success in Kip's class. Slowly, her teachers bought into her social thinking program and were willing to follow a slightly different path with Cait. I made my peace, too, and went beyond the walls of her high school for help. I signed Cait up at a highly regarded tutorial center. She worked with Liza, a wiry, red-headed woman with a love of language, a sense of humor, and a great way with my daughter. She quickly became another of Cait's prized knights, as she helped navigate assignments and stay in close touch with teachers. Twice a week throughout that winter, we trudged to the center late in the afternoon, no matter the weather. Cait never complained, even after a long day at school.

Late once on a frigid evening, after tutoring, Cait confided, "You know, Liza teaches me in a way I understand."

"That's wonderful." I let out a long exhale. After what felt like an eternity, Cait was finally getting what she needed in a way she could comprehend. I may have been busted, but darn it all, in the end, this one I got right.

22

HATS OFF

The day of Cait's high school graduation was warm and sunny—a good sign. I took the day off from work, my father flew in from New York, and Cait's great-aunt and dad drove up from Boston. Jay, who'd given her the "wrong" movie tape, showed up. Patrice, who had helped her navigate her thievery impulses during her Crafty Girl days arrived from Cape Cod, and of course, Courtney, Sam, Mike, and I were there with bells on, actually New Year's Eve noisemakers. This was one occasion those of us who loved Cait were not going to miss.

Weeks earlier, Cait and I, along with her knights—the teachers and specialists who worked with her as a senior—sat around a table one last time for her transition meeting. Our battles had come to an end. It was time to call a truce, or at least so I'd thought. Her English teacher, Mr. Dunn, who'd questioned the path I encouraged Cait to take, a two-year college program for students with learning challenges, now asked, "How are you feeling about going away to school in the fall, Cait?"

"Excited." Good answer.

"What do you think will challenge you the most?" Seriously?

"Well, I guess living away from home."

I didn't know what else he was expecting. Wouldn't any other graduating student report those very same feelings? Or was he banking on Cait to bail? "I don't really want to go!" With tears streaming down her face, Cait points a finger, "She's making me!"

It didn't happen.

Her learning specialist offered her congratulations, "Cait, we're really proud of you."

"I know," Cait grinned.

But Mr. Dunn, however, wasn't ready to acquiesce, "Cait, college *will* be different. You won't have the same help you had here." Check.

My turn. "*Actually*, it's a school for students with learning challenges. Everyone there needs assistance on some level." Checkmate.

"That's great." He shifted his comment back to Cait, "Are you ready for this new responsibility?"

"Yes," Cait and I chimed in together.

I'd been both admonished and applauded at Cait's school. At times I drove a hard bargain, and other times not nearly hard enough. I didn't always get her what she needed, but they couldn't fault me for not trying, or say I wasn't there for my daughter. So what if teachers argued I helped Cait do things she couldn't accomplish on her own. In the end, I helped my daughter soar. I wasn't just a helicopter parent all these years, I was her wingman, and now I was asking her to fly solo.

But what were my other options? If I didn't believe in my daughter, who would? I knew keeping her home would squelch any chances for independence. We lived in a rural place. The local community college was more than ten miles away and Cait didn't drive. She'd have to make friends with students who commuted from work. She needed to be in a place where a social life and friendships could happen for her.

If I showed my hand at the table, everyone sitting around it would have known I was as worried as they were about Cait living away from home and managing her classes without a traveling companion, even in a place designed for students with special needs. There was one thing, however, I was sure about. Cait needed this chance to continue on her trajectory. I couldn't predict where she'd land, but I knew that without challenging her and pushing her to move forward, she wouldn't get very far.

I faced my adversaries one last time and smiled, "I think Cait's going to be just fine."

As the sun slowly descended on that early summer evening, it was easy to enjoy its afterglow and to celebrate the class of 2009's journey. Chairs were set up facing the seventy-five graduates. The junior class would lead them down the steep steps in front of the school and across the wide lawn. Once seated, the graduates would look back out on their audience and on the school where they had grown and changed over the years.

I remembered when the decision was made for Cait to have an extra high school year. We had all agreed it would give Cait more time to mature and less of a course load. I insisted Cait not have to march out twice as a junior and sit through two long ceremonies. Everyone agreed, so she marched the year before, leading those students that would have been her graduating class. I wondered then if she regretted not being with them. She had to sit for a long stretch listening to endless awards and speeches. Often in those situations she'd fiddle, noticeably stretch, clear her throat, do practically anything to keep herself from bursting out of her chair. When I finally dropped her off to fill her duty as a junior, I had intended simply to watch her march out. Then I would leave, returning afterward to pick her up. But the evening was beautiful, so I stayed. Occasionally, I'd glance in her direction. She sat erect in her chair and stared serenely ahead. I couldn't detect one out-of-place movement. Occasionally, our eyes would meet and we'd smile. "Who is this child?" I thought. Clearly, she was no longer a child. She'd turned a corner that I'd somehow missed. I felt certain that the next year she'd be ready for her own turn at center stage.

My favorite tradition at Cait's school was baccalaureate. The Sunday before Cait's graduation a service took place in the town's

226-year-old, white, clapboard church. Families were seated along the wooden pews as the class, dressed in caps and gowns, marched in to the church's organ. There were several readings, choral presentations, and a selected faculty member spoke. The soft lights and intimacy of the church kept the tone of the evening solemn and reflective. I watched Cait sit with her shoulders relaxed, several pews ahead of us, and wondered what she was thinking. Were her thoughts about what lay ahead or what she was leaving behind?

Several days later, on the lawn that stretched out in front of her school, I watched the wave of school colors march down the steps, two by two. When it was Cait's turn, she moved carefully, keeping in time with her partner. Shortly after being seated, the students were up again, following the tradition of delivering flowers as a way to say thanks to the people who'd helped them. They each collected their allotted, two white carnations from the plastic buckets lining the stage. Cait moved through the crowd until she found her sister and me. I realized right then I should have snuck her a dozen more. There were so many who'd played a part, big and small, to get Cait to where she was right now. Teachers, helpers, administrators, all struggled on the path with her, each in their own way. Though her grandfather, now in his late eighties, didn't always understand what set this young woman apart, he was her biggest supporter and unfailingly made sure I could afford her special tutorial programs. But the equation worked in both directions: It was safe to say, Cait had made an impact on all of us as well. The educational assistant who saw her through most of high school went on to become a learning specialist. Cait, she said, was her inspiration.

When awards and scholarships were being given out, I played out my own for Cait privately in my head: this one is for the girl who would save one animal at a time; this one is for the girl who got herself to school each day, no matter how hard, and gave it her best.

When Cait's name was called to walk up and receive her diploma, we stood and cheered with our noisemakers while I dashed along the side to take her picture. Our Cait had done it.

When it finally ended, dusk had settled. We moved through the crowd until we found her and her classmates under a string of white lights where families and friends moved along, offering congratulations. In each photo we took, Cait was beaming. The woman who had worked with Cait for so many years brought her a bouquet adorned with an orange and black monarch butterfly; how fitting for the girl who had finally left her chrysalis.

As the crowd started to dwindle, I asked Cait if she was ready to rejoin her classmates. "Do you want to change for Project Graduation? The bus will be leaving soon." After months of fundraising, parents were providing a safe place for all the graduates to gather and celebrate together. Shortly after the ceremony a bus would whisk them away to an area health club where activities were planned. The bus would bring them back early the next day.

Cait hugged everyone goodbye and walked with me to where I had parked the car.

I passed over her bag. "Give me your cap and gown. I think you've got everything you need in the bag."

"I'm keeping the cap." Of course, she was the hat girl. I couldn't help but smile. Everyone was meeting up in the school's gym. "Have you got your yearbook to have people sign?"

"Yup."

"Okay, graduate. Have a great time. I'm really proud of you."

We hugged and then she walked up the steps to the gym as a classmate held open the door.

The rest of our family had already driven back to the house. Mike waited to drive back with me. As we were pulling into the driveway my cell phone rang. It was Cait.

"Hi, what's up?"

"Can you take me home?"

I glanced over at Mike. "Seriously?" She hadn't even left the parking lot.

"I'm tired. I really don't want to go."

"Okay, I'll come right up." I shook my head. "She didn't last five minutes."

"It's her night. When you see her, don't say a word." Mike got out and I swung the car around.

Crowds were still mingling here and there, as I parked and walked toward the gym. I found her waiting right inside the gym door where I'd last seen her. "Are you sure you don't want to go and spend the night with your classmates?"

"I'm sure." She was already heading outside toward the car.

I was disappointed; it was her last opportunity to be part of her class. But, I followed Mike's advice, and didn't try to convince her otherwise. She lived her life on the fringe. Why should this night be different? It was Cait's evening to shine and take center stage, to feel comfortable and happy. She wouldn't get that in a noisy bus or in a health club, locked in until the wee hours of the morning.

As we turned into the driveway, our house stood, like a beacon, lit up and filled with familiar faces. As Cait raced into the house, I could hear her sister, "Hey, grad. We're chowing down your cake. You'd better get some before it's all gone."

We crowded around the kitchen leaning against the counters with plates of Cait's favorite chocolate cake, smothered in butter cream frosting. Her sister raised her dish. Cait and the rest of us followed.

"Hip, hip, hooray!"

"You did it, Cait!"

"Way to go, girl!"

And with that, Cait took her tasseled cap, and tossed it up in the air.

Part III

DANCE UPON THE MOUNTAINS

"Faeries, come take me out of this dull world,
For I would ride with you upon the wind,
Run on the top of the disheveled tide,
And dance upon the mountains like a flame."

Poet W.B. Yeats, *The Land of Heart's Desire*

23

THE LAUNCH

Before Cait headed off to college, you couldn't be around me without getting caught up in my frenzy to launch Cait on her next adventure—unless you were Cait, who did a good job of remaining oblivious. Maybe I should have taken her lack of involvement as a sign. Or at least begged the question and asked myself if Cait was really prepared for this next step. I didn't.

No matter where we were that summer, it was all about getting ready.

"When we're in New York visiting your grandfather, we're checking out Ikea."

"I . . . what?" She gazed up from her Minecraft game while still playing. How does she do that?

"A place where we can get all kinds of things for your dorm room." I, at least, was pumped.

"Nice." This time she didn't even give a look my way, but I didn't care. These were those college gates I had been waiting for. I was determined not to have a failed launch. I had enough of those as Cait was growing up leading to my own version of PTSD: early departures from summer camp, after-school programs that didn't fly, volunteer jobs that didn't work out. I refused to entertain anything but her success, so I consumed myself with endless lists like the proverbial mother of the bride.

A couple of weeks later, I was walking with Cait through the automatic doors of Ikea, the Swedish version of "If we don't have it, you don't need it."

"Will you look at this place!" I was hoping some of my enthusiasm would transfer over to my daughter.

"You know he said I could have a fish." Cait was replaying her conversation with the dean who had interviewed her. In a store where they had just about everything imaginable, Cait was thinking about the one thing they didn't have—pets. I chose to ignore the comment. "Let's head to the bedding."

While I was painstakingly color coordinating her sheets and comforters, I found Cait in the next department draped over an imitation white fur rug.

"This is perrrrrfect," she purred.

While I was elated over locating a lamp and wastebasket that matched her blanket, she delighted in finding bamboo plants next to housewares. I made her tag along after me through Ikea's towering warehouse aisles as I looked for a chair, finally spying one on the second level. I visualized her curled up in its soft cushion, reading and studying on chilly nights. It was the image I clung to as we headed through the checkout.

As if dragging her to Ikea for furniture wasn't enough, I tortured her even more with endless runs to Staples and Walmart, where we acquired every imaginable office supply. While she was searching for a Hello Kitty binder, I sneaked extra highlighters and sticky notes into the cart. I purchased containers, and more containers—just in case. I organized and labeled and packed. I loaded up her shower caddy with herbal shampoos, cream rinse, bar soap, body wash, fragrant lotions, razors—blessed with my mantra, "Don't forget to shave your legs"—and finally a pink loofah. The caddy could have sunk a small boat, but if she went down, at least she'd be clean. The corner in our living room designated as "Cait's college holding tank" grew exponentially on a daily basis.

I wasn't naïve enough to think that college was all about office supplies and perfectly sized sheets. I also made sure that Cait continued to work with her writing tutor twice a week, although she'd much rather have been swimming. I labeled her weekly pillbox and lost sleep over where she should keep it so as not to forget her all-important daily dose of attention meds and mood stabilizers. I gained enough organizational knowledge to become a wedding planner and enough nervous energy to become bridezilla.

When her departure day finally arrived, Cait suddenly exhibited her well-hidden elation while I developed my own rapid heartbeat. I didn't bother going back over my endless lists because there wasn't a spare inch left in the car for anything I might have forgotten. Her school was just a little over an hour south of our house. I think its close proximity made both of us breathe a little easier. Her sister's trip to college years earlier had taken six hours.

Arrival on campus was a blur. We had to first maneuver an endless maze of stations in the gymnasium—college ID, laundry service, clubs, tech support—before they'd let Cait begin her new life. It was crowded and stuffy and the lines endless. If she didn't bail here with the noise level and confusion, she'd be okay, at least for the next twelve hours.

I started scanning the room like a hawk, pushing her through the stations that seemed to matter most. I was itching to get to her dorm room, to unload and organize her life for the next nine months, and to size up her roommate, the stranger that could make or break her first college semester away from home—that and about a million other things.

Finally, we were driving to the cinder block dormitory furthest up the hill, having chosen the dorm months earlier because of its extended quiet hours. Murphy's Law dictated that hers would be the room on the second story, down an endless hallway. Her roommate was already settling in, but not without her own anxious parents and older sister. Avery was small and delicate, but her athletic shorts and team t-shirt screamed sports as did the one and only poster (of a soccer-playing girl) above her bed. Cait couldn't be more different from the girl she was about to set up house next to. After brief introductions, I was glad to escape and begin our own countless trips to the car. I dripped sweat and Cait moaned as we lifted and dragged the contents of the car into her cramped space, yet her fussing was a lot less than I would have suspected. I suppose that to her, each heavy box meant one step closer to freedom.

Following each drop-off, we'd pause long enough to exchange polite small talk. Her roommate turned out to be from Maryland. With a car full of passengers, they had under-packed and were stressing about Vermont's first snow. Although they hadn't managed to fit all of Avery's winter gear into the trunk, there had still been enough room in the car for her microwave, TV and Wii, which she generously offered up to Cait anytime she had the inclination. While Avery's parents had images of a shivering daughter trudging through mounds of white in tennis shoes, the images of Cait that crowded my mind were far worse—of Cait plugged in, while her books piled up collecting dust. Already I was afraid it wasn't going to work.

Avery's dad, left standing around while his wife and daughters worked, engaged in polite conversation with us, while we made Cait's bed and stuffed clothes into her tiny closet. "So, what are you called if you live in Vermont?"

"Vermonter," I responded with my biggest "Vermonter" grin.

"Really?" he mused, "How about if you're from New Hampshire?"

"New Hampshirerite." My smile was fading.

"Fancy that," he chuckled and went on.

Was he serious? I wondered if I'd have to go through all fifty states. So he was a Trivial Pursuit buff, but what about his daughter and what brought her here?

Avery's mom suddenly announced a much-needed trip to Walmart and before I could blink, they all walked out, leaving Cait and me alone in her room. Should I have been the one to initiate a discussion about our daughters? Admittedly, it felt awkward, but no more than what we were asking our kids to do: Share sleeping quarters with a complete stranger.

When we first arrived, Avery confided that she'd been to college before, but it didn't work out. I wondered what challenges overwhelmed her? Did she harbor any quirks or idiosyncrasies? Cait had a long list of them. I would have happily shared, even a few of her quirks, but I missed my chance as they disappeared down the hall.

Once I was satisfied Cait was settled in, I dragged her to every meeting on our orientation itinerary. The president's welcome speech, under a large white, billowing tent in the middle of the soccer field, reminded me of one of those picture-perfect wedding days, sunny and cloud free. It's hard not to believe this union couldn't be anything but flawless. Surely success will await Cait around every corner here. Several students shared their personal challenges and achievements. One young man joked about his wandering attention; a flittering butterfly across the field could pull him a mile off course. Cait laughed. She understood. Maybe it was only a well-planned sales pitch, but if they had served Kool-Aid, I would have downed several glasses.

After, Cait went off to a student meeting on the other side of campus, while I followed a wave of parents headed for the fine arts building. I kept glancing back until she was lost in the crowd, hoping she'd be okay. When I got to the assembly hall, it was packed. My favorite seat, last row at the end of the aisle, where I could sneak out unnoticed, was already taken. I ended up in the front center with a perfect view of the stage and the assembled staff ready to explain programs and services. As I sat there, I could physically feel the adrenaline level rise on all sides. If there had been a stress barometer, it would have read "approaching storm." Administraton and faculty members barely finished their introductions when questions were fired from the audience.

"What's the system for communicating grades?"

"How do students navigate services?"

"What support systems will help my son stay on track?"

The panel tried to field the barrage of questions, often deferring to the other. I felt their distress mixing with my own, and I began to squirm in my seat. The dean finally conceded, "As students adjust to living away from home, the first term can often be muddy." Muddy? It was the wrong answer for this audience and it fueled more questions. Though I understood their panic, I realized the group on stage couldn't guarantee success. I no longer cared that I was dead center; I got up and made my escape.

I finally caught up with Cait at the dining hall. At the very least, the school put out a decent spread resembling a Thanksgiving dinner, but in late August. As we maneuvered to an open table, I spotted Avery with her dad and several other athletic types. I hadn't seen him at any of the parent meetings. Walmart must have had long lines that day. I never had the chance to explain away some of Cait's behaviors or her one-way conversations. It wouldn't be until a few weeks later, and a visit from Courtney, that Cait's differences would be explained to Avery and an open invitation to Courtney's Facebook page in case questions cropped up.

Unlike high school, college was the best place I knew for students just a shade different from their peers. Besides opportunities to learn and explore, there'd be other kindred spirits on Cait's wavelength. In the end, Avery wasn't one of them and moved out half way through the year to be with a friend. But the two did find one bit of common ground that first semester—*Grey's Anatomy* on Thursday nights.

24

MUDDY WATERS

When Cait first went off to college, I didn't expect miracles, but I admit to praying for greater independence. My biggest worry, living away from home for the first time, seemed to come easiest for her. She loved her freedom—from me, from her ed assistants, from any and all imposed rules or expectations. She relished making her own decisions. Unfortunately, when she was making those decisions, she didn't always take into consideration the main reason she was there—her classes.

To be fair, given the profusion of safety nets in Cait's life prior to college, she wasn't going to instantly morph into an independent and motivated scholar, but I was hoping she would at least make a start.

"Cait, did you connect with your advisor?"

"Not yet. Every time I go, she's with someone."

"You really need to get in to see her." A feeling of worry took root in my chest, one that wouldn't be displaced.

Miraculously, Cait made it through her first four days of orientation. I would have thought it would have included a face-to-face with the advisor, the point person who'd hopefully come to know

Cait inside and out, figure out her weaknesses, and be there to catch her before she stumbled. When I realized I was describing myself, I decided that maybe Cait didn't need an advisor as much as I had thought. Still, I would have liked at least a "Hello, nice to meet you," from the woman. It didn't happen.

By the end of week two, whenever I had a break at work, I found myself headed for a picnic bench just outside the faculty room, where I had cell reception. I had started a phone list of school personnel who could explain to me why my daughter's advisor seemed to have disappeared into thin air. I couldn't believe the term had begun and Cait hadn't even met her yet. They assured me they were on it.

By week three I was on the phone to her sister. "Okay, it's probably not too cool for me to show up at her school like some lunatic mother demanding, 'Who the hell is my daughter's advisor and why hasn't she connected with my kid yet?' So you do it. Then take your sister out to dinner. It's on me." A grilled burger or slice of pizza on the fly wasn't much payment for yet another imposed sisterly act of kindness, but I was desperate.

I figured Courtney, a recent psychology graduate, with years of camp counselor experience and employment at a college mentoring program, possessed the right amount of savvy to get things in motion. And better than any of that, she loved her sister and wanted things to go well.

Late one afternoon, she drove from her home in southern New Hampshire to her sister's campus. The plan was to corner the advisor and embarrass her into seeing Cait on the spot. The prior lack of connection on both ends was plain crazy. It was like some sort of kamikaze mission and we all knew who'd be the one to crash and burn. Cait was a master at avoidance, but this same trait coming from her advisor was inconceivable to me, especially from such a high profile school, one that liked to boast of their achievements through continual radio advertisements.

For one afternoon, Courtney became me, the Black Hawk. Her mission, sweep down and target the one person who could save Cait her first semester. Amazingly, she found her and made the introductions. As the advisor and Cait stepped into her office, Courtney, who had learned from a lifetime of watching me, positioned herself just within earshot of the closed door.

"So, Caitlin, how are things going?"

"Fine."

"That's wonderful."

That's it?

As Cait exited, Courtney informed the woman that her sister hadn't accessed any of the school's resources and she was therefore going to help familiarize her with a few of them. My twenty-something-year-old daughter was doing her job.

Courtney dragged her sister to the study center, then to the coaching department, signing her up along the way. She even went back to her dorm room to meet the roomie and take them both out to dinner. She did all a sister could do.

Though Courtney helped to get the advisor relationship established, Cait was still vague about what was expected. I worried she was a sinking ship that had barely left the harbor. Her first weeks already reflected some missed classes as she got days and times confused, and her assignments weren't registering. I began to doubt she followed through on the initial appointments her sister set up. When Cait had entered this specialized school, I had been hopeful that I would be passing the torch to her next set of guardian angels, the ones that were something akin to patron saints. I figured there must be one for all college-bound Asperger's kids. I inwardly promised I'd pray to him or her every night, just as long as it let me off the hook and I didn't have to once again help her navigate school.

Those thoughts never left my mind, even after I established my new Saturday morning ritual, driving an hour south and sitting next to Cait in the hard plastic bucket chairs at the local Laundromat. I'd pump quarters into the machines and would return to sit next to her as she balanced her English notebook on one knee. "So, what's your assignment this week?"

"I need to write about myself for my Learning Perspectives class. You know, something I've learned, but what makes it hard for me. I need to describe a situation, but I can't think of any."

Seriously? I could write a book. Would your teacher like the long version or just a single-spaced, ten-page synopsis with nine-point font! "Hmm, sounds like an interesting assignment, Cait. I'm sure we can brainstorm *something*."

It would take until the clothes were all laundered and folded for Cait to scratch out some of her thoughts. Often times, while I listened to her t-shits and jeans thumping around in rhythmic circles, I'd be her scribe, pulling out enough words for a page that she could then later type. I knew that her school was considered the premier place for students with learning challenges. What I didn't understand was why I was in the Laundromat on Saturday mornings. I had assumed theirs was going to be a foolproof method for catching the kids who were struggling. Students would learn how to set about tackling assignments. When I thought back on that first parent meeting in late summer, I imagined this is what the dean meant when he talked about muddy waters. Good thing we found the Laundromat.

25

LEARNING CURVE

Parent weekend couldn't have come too soon. I was finally going to meet the MIA advisor and get a better sense of what was truly going on at the start of Cait's first term. I took a personal day from work so I could be there for all three days.

Late that second afternoon, Cait led me down a flight of stairs to the basement of an old brick building. Two chairs were waiting for us in the hallway outside her advisor's office. I could hear voices on the other side of the door. It sounded like a parent with her son. I tried to catch the flavor of their conversation. I didn't consider it eavesdropping as much as learning if maybe they, too, were members of the Muddy Waters Club.

When their time was up, we were ushered in. As I sat opposite Cait's advisor, I quickly scanned the space. There was no desk, just two long tables squaring off one corner of her room. Above one were high windows where sunlight was replaced by feet walking by. On the table below were some toys, semi-adult ones, if you stretched it—cube puzzles, squishy balls, all the things that attention deficient kids would glom onto, even eighteen- to twenty-something-year-olds. There was one organizer with lots of forms, but most of her paperwork waited in piles, some spreading out onto the floor. The lone bookshelf was bulging with books and folders. Two brass hooks held a black robe and sash, probably there since last year's graduation.

Was this really the woman who'd teach her advisees how to get organized? On the wall beyond her was an elaborate word bank, holding close to two hundred words or more. So you teach English. Her waist length hair and long flowing skirt suggested that she and I came from the same Woodstock generation, but she still dressed for the festival.

"Hi, Cait. How are you?!" She was friendly and outgoing, which seemed to put Cait at ease. That part I liked. She swung her chair back around to face her computer and began pulling up Cait's records. "So Cait, how do you think things are going?" she asked over her shoulder.

"I don't know. I guess okay."

After a few minutes of friendly chatter, she dove into Cait's new reality—she wasn't okay, more like, overwhelmed. Four classes was an overload. Cait agreed to drop her history class, currently her lowest grade, figuring F was as low as she could go. The rest hovered right above it. The wilderness survival class she was taking for PE was a pass/fail, but her performance there was dicey.

"Cait, your teacher reports that you're having a hard time staying focused. You seem to have a lot of displaced energy. It's a distraction. Can you put a finger on what's happening?" Every time she spoke to Cait, she ended her sentence with a nervous laugh. It was starting to irritate me.

"Sometimes I drink a Red Bull. I guess I'm eating a lot of other junk too."

"That can do it Cait," I chimed in, "Don't do it anymore, okay?"

Her advisor laughed again, as though she'd heard it all before. I wasn't finding humor in any of it.

I hadn't taken my eyes off Cait, "Where can you go for help?"

"Well, there's the study center and the academic support center."

I knew that Cait had finally made it over to the study center. "How's that going Cait?"

"Okay, but sometimes it's hard to concentrate."

She had shown me the place as we toured around that day. On the lower level of one of the dorms was a room with cubicles. Similar to a high school study hall, it was staffed in the afternoons and offered students assistance with their assignments. It wasn't ideal.

"What about the academic support center, Cait?" I suddenly realized I was asking all the questions.

"Okay, I'll try it."

Students had to sign up where the sessions were held. Somehow, I didn't see Cait grabbing the bull by the horns and being that organized. The faculty was assigned tutoring slots, which changed on a daily basis. Cait would never have the same person. It would be like visiting a foreign country, each time hoping they understood your dialect. This wasn't going to work. I left her advisor's office feeling a little like I, too, was mucking around in the mud.

Cait needed to get out of the hole she was in, so I continued to drive down on weekends, helping her pass her first term's assignments.

I never threw away the school's personnel list of phone numbers and continued to make my pitch to anyone who'd listen. Cait needed a "go-to," someone to help with all the executive functioning that wasn't happening. Someone who would make sure she understood her assignments, help her manage her time, set deadlines, advise her on a tutor, and maybe even proof her work. I was told that advisors could do what I was suggesting. They scheduled her for two meetings weekly with the lady in the basement.

Cait's second term had to go better. She adjusted to life away from home and now had a vague awareness of what was expected. Her advisor had signed her up for some favorite classes: biology, photography, a required English course that focused on environmental issues, history, and yoga.

Two weeks in, we realized, once again, four academic classes were over her limit. Again, history was dropped. Cait would never become a historian, but she was immersed now in subjects that she had always loved, and she appeared happy. When I asked her about a class, she reported back that things were going great.

I guess the Kool-Aid I sipped under the big white, billowing tent months earlier was finally kicking in. I believed this was Cait's turning point, but I didn't completely let my guard down. Some weekends I coaxed Cait to come home so we could check on things together.

"In English we have a research paper. I'm doing mine on the destruction of tropical rainforests and what it means for the world."

"Perfect topic, Cait."

She pulled out of her pack lots of books on the subject. I pulled out a pack of index cards and an old high school research paper she had done for a history class to use as a model.

"Remember this, Cait? It's a good template. Use the note cards to keep track of your resources."

"I'm on it." She sounded sincere.

When I asked about biology, she smiled. "It's going great." This was her new mantra; everything was always great. I'd ask her about labs, and she assured me she was on those, too.

I had no reason to doubt her. Her school had a system for keeping parents in the loop. Each week students and advisors met to go over their current grades and class standing. Absences were noted, as was missing or late work, and teacher comments were made. If a student was in trouble, they received a warning and their advisor was notified. A second warning was sent home alerting parents. During Cait's entire spring I never received a warning. I was lulled into thinking that Cait was actually doing okay, but more than that, I desperately wanted to believe it. Maybe it was my desperation that made me fail to notice the warning signs.

When Cait was home for March break, I encouraged her to keep working on her research paper for English. Her index cards were filling up. I glanced in her notebook and found a paper with some writing that wasn't hers. "What's this, Cait?"

"Oh that's when I went to the study center and got help." Help consisted of a brief outline of ideas for her paper adding up to no more that about five lines.

"This is great, Cait, but it's just a start. Let's add to it." I knew what she currently had in front of her wasn't going to come close to producing an entire paper.

Her photography class was becoming more and more of a challenge for her. The class that she thought was all about taking pictures was more about developing them and using a variety of speeds and exposures. That April, during a three-day break, we visited her grandfather. We headed out to the Long Island beaches and she took a bunch of pictures that would need developing. "Is this the only thing required?"

"Yes, now all I need is more time in the dark room." I knew she wasn't going to be the next Ansel Adams, but she seemed okay.

In high school her favorite classes had been in science, so I didn't ask to see her lab reports for her biology class. I believed at the very least, she was managing her work there. Yes! This is what college is supposed to look like.

About a month before the term was ending, Cait had a mini meltdown. She broke down crying in her advisor's office. She couldn't be consoled, nor could she put a finger on what was troubling her: overload, stress, a long winter? Her advisor walked her over to the counseling center and emailed her instructors telling them Cait was especially fragile right now. I was beginning to appreciate the woman's low-key manner and her sensitivity to Cait's emotional needs.

It seemed like we were in the home stretch, and then, the bottom fell out. A week before finals her advisor emailed me. "Cait's passing, but only barely."

I immediately wrote her back. "You're telling me this one week before the end of the term? What am I suppose to do now? Where are my parent warnings?"

I couldn't believe it. Cait had come home to prep for finals. I figured it was her only shot to pull everything back up. I couldn't do much about photography, but I had her work her tail off on her research paper for English. As I went through her notes, I kept looking for the work leading up to her final report. Where were the outlines? All I could find was the scribbled, skeletal one someone had scratched out in the study center earlier. "Cait, this can't be all your work. There must be more." This class was supposed to lay the groundwork for all future papers. "Didn't he give you a list of assignments?"

That's when I learned about their campus website where instructors posted their requirements. Though some gave paper copies, most only posted. And that's where I found the work leading up to the final report. It was ironic to me that her advisor, a fellow English instructor, never mentioned this. She must have known the format used in the freshman English class. Cait now had to work backwards.

Since I didn't receive any notices from the grade reporting system, I hoped we had prevented Cait from another crash before the end of her second semester. She came home at the end of her first year and waited for her final grades.

A week later an envelope arrived in our post-office box. I got in the car and handed it over to her. "And the winner is . . ." I bantered as we exited the parking lot.

She smiled back and quickly tore it open scanning the page. "Oh, my God. I can't believe I did this badly."

I glanced over. I was convinced she was teasing me.

"I got an F in biology and Ds in everything else!"

This had to be a joke. She was really playing it up. I watched her complete her biology final at home, and she reported to have done the labs. How could she have gotten an F? "Cait, you're kidding, right?"

"No, I'm not. I'm dead serious."

I pulled the car over alongside the road and read the paper now lying open in her lap. She was serious. For the first time, we were both on the same page, stunned and speechless. I had not received a warning from any of her instructors, nor from their fancy system.

Muddy water? No, this was quicksand. Cait was up to her neck and quickly disappearing down to the bottom.

She turned to me. "Hey, I passed yoga."

I looked up, "Yeah, Cait. You've officially mastered the downward-facing dog."

26

SCENE ONE, TAKE TWO

Failing grades were not what I had envisioned when Cait went off to college. It wasn't how I wanted her to end her first year. I didn't know whether to be pissed or devastated. I did know that the only way I could sleep at night was to get down to Cait's school and figure out what had gone wrong. Even more pressing, I needed to know what would happen to Cait's scholarship money for the following fall term now that she was officially below a 2.0 grade point average. Once again, I pulled out the now well-worn list of "go-to" personnel and made the call to the head of advising. The following week, with Cait waiting in the hallway, I was sitting opposite him. I was armed with every email from my inbox. Not one of them remotely suggested that Cait was in the F zone in any of her classes. He pulled up the semester's grade reports along with the end-of-the-term comments. Each one applauded Cait's attendance, but at the same time said she was either missing work, or had handed it in too late. It appeared that her "everything's fine" biology class was missing numerous labs. I'm not sure what planet she was on when she said they were completed.

"I don't understand it. If she was doing so poorly in that class, why was I never sent a warning? For that matter, I didn't receive warnings for any of her classes."

The first-year academic dean had joined us. She, along with the head advisor, looked over at me sheepishly. "Well," continued the head of advising, "She didn't start doing poorly until near the end of the term."

"That often happens to students," the first-year dean commented. "They begin to bottom out as they move into finals."

I wasn't buying it. I pulled out the pathetic outline for her English paper done at their study center. "This was the help she got at the study center. Didn't someone take a look at her other work to see where she was in the process?" They couldn't answer me. "She can't have the same academic advisor next term. It's not working. Cait was seriously floundering and she didn't pick up on it."

I gave them my now patent speech about "what she really needs is the nonexistent point person to help her figure out assignments." I knew exactly what was happening and why their system wasn't working. Cait would show up for her advisor meeting and would be asked how things were going. She'd report back, "Just fine," and would leave.

She needed someone who would tell her to open up the notebook and show them what "just fine" looked like. But I still couldn't understand why their reporting system didn't signal Cait's academic advisor how dire her situation had become.

"Who signs up an Asperger's kid for photography anyway? It was like signing her up to speak Russian. Cait thought she was going to be taking some pictures and doing a little developing, but the class was all about different exposures and shutter speeds. There was no way on God's Earth she could have kept track of that stuff."

The first-year dean commiserated with me. "I agree. I had another student like Cait who couldn't manage it either." I could sense she knew exactly what I was talking about, but it was after the fact. What is it that they say about hindsight? It wasn't going to help Cait.

"You know," she went on, "We have a policy at our school that you can retake a class that you've failed and if you pass, it will replace the F."

I politely listened as my own monologue ran rampant in my head. Cait, will never graduate this place. There's no way she can redo an entire term.

We all agreed to change her current academic advisor. The head of advising conveniently needed to leave for another meeting. Before exiting, he threw a crumb my way by acknowledging my dilemma. "I know what you're saying. Our population here is changing and Cait, along with students like her, don't fit into our current model of services. We're trying to address it. Please make your concerns known when you speak to the provost."

He's my next stop.

Cait and I stayed and worked with the first-year academic dean to switch around classes for the next fall. She seemed to have a handle on instructors who would match Cait's learning profile and her interests. Cait was going to retake biology, but not the other classes. She could withstand a couple of Ds as long as she began passing her new classes and raising her grade point average.

The provost had pat answers for all my concerns. He assured me Cait's money would be there in the fall, provided that she passed her classes the following term. He also told me one big, whopping lie. When I described the perfect advisor for someone like Cait, he assured me that there was enough flexibility within their advisor program to meet the needs of individual students in the way that made sense for them. If that were true, he must have been spending most of his time on planet Cait.

27

PRACTICE MAKES PERFECT
(or Close Enough)

I remember it like yesterday. It was Cait's first summer home from college. She and I were crossing the Whitestone Bridge from Queens, Long Island, heading home to Vermont, after visiting family. Cars were at a stand still leaving me to look over at the post-9/11 skyline. I heard what sounded like a buzzer. The windows were down to let in the warm air as well as ward off my claustrophobia. When the exhaust fumes started to replace the fresh air, I rolled them back up, hearing the noise again. It was coming from inside the car. "What's that sound?" Cait was intently looking at the screen on her phone. "A text."

A what? Prior thoughts of terrorists holding hundreds of cars hostage on the bridge were replaced with one thought only, Cait's got a friend! I had trouble containing myself.

"So," I exhaled slowly, "Who's the message from?"

"Just someone at school."

Before I could shoot off another question, cars started moving. The whole while we crawled through the tollbooth, her phone beeped and her fingers scrambled over the keys in response. Once the traffic sped up, I resumed my questioning, while waves of euphoria washed over me at the thought of Cait actually making a social connection.

"What's this person's name?"

"Nicole."

"Was she in your classes?"

"No, I see her and her boyfriend in the cafeteria. I call him Blue Boy, because his hair is dyed blue."

"Oh, cool." Did I really just say that? I refused to pass judgment. She was communicating, which was all that mattered.

"But, I'm not texting her anymore, this is someone else."

Am I dreaming? "How are their summers going? Will they be returning to school in the fall?"

No response. Her grin widened as she read a new message. I felt like I had just hit social media megabucks.

When Cait went off to college, I imagined her forging new friendships in the same fashion she parallel played as a child. Back then she never fully joined in, but she could still learn the nuances of the game from her place along the sidelines. This way she could set her own rules and there was no pressure. She was a participant without participating. It met her social needs then, so why not now? Yet, on the other hand, a lot had changed since her days of Legos and sand castles. My role, however, always remained the same—the anxious parent hoping her daughter would achieve social success. I figured there must be someone out there who shared her interests and appreciated her young spirit and offhanded humor.

Now that she was in college, I couldn't rely on teachers to satisfy my curiosity with progress reports or occasional phone calls, so Cait fell victim to my daily inquisitions.

"Anyone interesting in your classes?"

"Who'd you eat dinner with last night?"

"Do you think you'll eat with them again tonight?"

She was a saint for not hanging up on me. Occasionally, I was rewarded with an actual classmate's name, something she was never good at remembering. Though Cait seemed to spend a lot of time in her dorm room, she appeared happy with college life. While I was aware that some of her classmates struggled with the college's rural setting, Cait remained content. If she was home on the weekend, she was always eager to go back, but I never sensed there were friends awaiting her return.

That summer my "friendship worries" took a turn. Cait's phone was on constant vibrate, with one boy in particular, Cim, who lived in Florida. Occasionally, Cait would talk on the phone to him, but primarily her communication was via cryptic messages across a tiny phone screen. I could quickly tell that Cim, like Cait, enjoyed a lot of the same interests, including posting art on a popular website and endless online chats. At the end of the summer, Cim sent her a large Hello Kitty stuffy. She was thrilled and I was amazed. Cim moved up to boyfriend status. I took her to buy a large bag of Sour Patch candy, Cim's favorite, for when they returned to school.

Once back, Cim never seemed to be part of the group she reported eating dinner with, though she shared they'd listen to music back in her room. On the surface, their relationship appeared like any other adolescent romance—moments of smooth sailing and occasional waves.

"How's Cim, Cait?"

"Okay, I haven't talked to him a lot lately."

"Why?"

"He's too busy."

"Are you okay with that?"

"Sure."

She seemed to weather the dynamics of their relationship well until one day several weeks into the new term. I was on campus for a meeting with her newest advisor. Cait was supposed to catch up with me after her class. As soon as I spotted her across the campus green, I knew something was wrong. By the time she reached me, tears were rolling down her cheeks. Cim had broken up with her. It had something to do with schoolwork.

I hugged her and we plopped right down on the grass as I proceeded to provide a long list of her sister's previous breakups adding a few of the gorier details for effect. "You're now part of the 'I Got Dumped Club.' Everyone I know has been a member at least once."

Her tears had stopped and I reached over to give her a hug.

I was secretly amazed. The child I worried about never connecting to anyone outside close family members and teachers was now acting like any teenager. But I ached for her, too. I knew her poor resiliency and lack of perspective were still her biggest challenges.

A day later, she surprised me again.

"Have you spoken to Cim? He might explain why he can't hang out with you anymore." I figured if she understood his reasons, it might make it easier.

"No!"

"Okay, I just thought . . ."

She cut me off. "He told me he couldn't talk." She was adamant.

Here, her literal interpretation paid off. I pondered all the other love-struck girls who would have made themselves a nuisance trying to salvage their first love. I gave her kudos for taking the high road on this one.

Over those first weeks fresh after the breakup I couldn't help but wonder if she was feeling uncomfortable running into Cim. It was a small campus, though I remembered that Cim wasn't part of her cafeteria group.

"It's fine," she reported, "I rarely see him." I caught a slight change in her expression, but she promised me she was okay.

I didn't have to worry, as Cim didn't remain off her social radar for very long. Before I knew it, he was again her text buddy when she came home for a weekend. It appeared that he was back on track in his classes, and so throughout the remaining fall and winter, he maintained boyfriend status.

When Cait arrived home for winter break, the first shopping we did was the bookstore. She chose several science fiction books, his passion. We barely posted the package to Florida, where he lived with his parents and younger brother, when in the mail two necklaces arrived, one in the shape of a heart. Cait wore them constantly.

After returning to school, their relationship seemed steady, and Valentine's Day produced a teddy bear, which Cait packed along with her clothes anytime she came home. I couldn't help but ask myself, who was this sweet and endearing boy? I wanted to meet him.

On a Sunday return drive I decided to put it out there. "Do you think Cim can swing by while I'm dropping you off?" Minutes earlier she had been text messaging him. We were approaching the exit. The timing was perfect.

"Not now. He's too busy with schoolwork."

"Cait, he's been hanging out with you in the car for the last thirty minutes. What's five minutes more, just to say hello?"

"No, Mom." I knew that tone and I wasn't in the mood to push it. I reasoned Cim must be dealing with some of his own social insecurities.

We moved into March and spring break brought both sisters home at the same time. Courtney was now a graduate student and living in Portland, Maine. When she returned, the rhythm of the house changed. Her chocolate lab, Izze, was a ball of energy. Courtney would immediately cajole Cait into helping unleash some of it. Shopping was also always on their list. I loved how Courtney helped to guide some of Cait's clothing choices away from the mismatched eclectic-wear purchased at the local used clothing store near her college. Cait would even agree to watch her sister's choice of chick flicks from the local movie rental while they'd give each other manicures. Over the years they developed an easy relationship, bringing them closer. Cait saw her sister not only as her friend, but as her confidant.

So I wasn't totally surprised one morning when Courtney came into my room and gently closed the door. She held her finger up to her lips and in a hushed tone signaled that she had something to tell me. "Promise," she whispered, "you're not going to overreact. There's something you need to know, but you've got to swear you won't say a word."

"Okay, not a word." I always got a little pit in my stomach when some hidden secret was about to be revealed, but this one was about to exceed my expectations.

"Cim is not at college. He's never been at college. She met him online."

"Oh my God! You've got to be kidding me."

"Remember, you promised."

I didn't know whether to laugh or cry. I was stunned, shaken, and ticked off all at once. My own gullibility startled me, but then jolted me back to Cait's reality, which was her total comfort in cyberspace.

Cait had met Cim on a popular deviant art website. I didn't disagree that their relationship was as real as any other, but she'd never laid eyes on him. She had lied and kept it hidden for months. My mind was on overload with flashbacks and light bulbs going off all at once. Why couldn't I have figured this out?

"You can't tell her you know. She'll never trust me again," Courtney, sister-now-turned-informant, brought me back.

"What am I going to do?" I asked, more to myself than my oldest daughter.

"Look, I told you because you really needed to know. I explained to her about being safe. She's never going to meet him, but you can't say anything, otherwise she'll never tell me anything again."

She was right. "You've just landed yourself a new job, my personal stool pigeon. I want to know everything." Courtney rolled her eyes, but I knew she cared about her sister and would continue to feed me the information I needed to keep Cait safe.

The hardest part was living the charade, but even worse, was my lack of trust in everything Cait told me. Maybe all her friends were from the web. For all I knew, she ate alone in a corner of the dining hall every night without a single friend in sight.

Each time I heard Cim's name I cringed, but played the game. I carried a huge knot inside—disappointment and fear all tied up in my gut.

Yet on another level that surprised even me, I was proud of another Cait-milestone. She finally got theory of mind—the ability to know what another person might be thinking and why. She had started to put herself in someone else's shoes—mine. She knew exactly where my comfort zone was and how I would have reacted to her online relationship with Cim. She figured out what she needed to tell me to keep her secret going. She achieved what a lot of Asperger's kids spend years learning, and some never acquire. On some twisted level, I was proud of her accomplishment.

While the two of us were out walking one day, she finally confessed. Maybe, confiding in Courtney was her trial run before talking to me. After a while, the deception must have weighed on her. I was grateful I already had my chance to "over react" in private. She understood the concerns already voiced about Internet relationships.

I couldn't deny that I was happy to see Cait finally connecting socially, even romantically, with a group of her peers, even if it was in cyberspace. This was her parallel play, her test drive, before she was ready to join the game. We did have to curtail her computer use while she was at school by blocking some of her favorite sites since it was easy for her to lose all sense of time. She maintained a lot of her connections through Facebook, which I deemed a more acceptable form of online chatting.

Cim broke up with her again, but she took it more in stride the second time. I still worried that she wouldn't apply her newly developing social skills to her school life, but happily her connections with her peers and her classes appeared to be growing and changing throughout that spring—and every one of her new friends inhabited her real world.

28

RIGHT TURN OR LEFT?

Cait and I had an agreement. At the start of each new semester, I would drive down the first two weekends to check-in. Our conversations were always the same. "Cait, beginnings are important. You want to know what's coming your way and how to organize yourself."

I didn't need to remind her of the prior crash and burn, when we were less diligent. So just after 10:30 a.m. on the Saturday of the new fall term, with enough time for her to sleep in and eat breakfast (my one concession), I whisked her and her bulging backpack off to the local library. We walked in, eyed a table perfect for spreading out her laptop and notebooks, and my inquisition began. "Okay, show me everything."

"Alright, alright," she'd grimace.

I knew other mothers who emptied their adolescents' backpacks for signs of illegal substances. Not something I worried about with Cait, though she dressed the part—laced black leather boots, ripped jeans, low cut t-shirt, dangling earrings, very Goth, very Cait . . . except for the face, all young and innocent. Hardly a match.

Long ago I discovered that parenting Cait was a little like driving on a freeway. Whenever I thought it was safe to put the car into cruise control, flashing orange lights on a big, bold sign warned: Major Roadwork Ahead.

I shouldn't have been too surprised to find myself that morning face-to-face with an already missed assignment. Even after my painstaking efforts to make sure she was up-to-date, I hadn't foreseen she'd miss her first field biology trip. Her excuse—a light drizzle.

"I can't believe you. Don't you get how important these trips are?"

No comment.

"You're a nature girl for God's sake." Did she miss the obvious or was she willful?

I'm not sure if it was meant as a punishment or an effort to save her, but the following Sunday afternoon, the two of us were hiking up the trail of Black Mountain in search of glacial deposits and tree succession. As the trail grew steeper, I peeked over my shoulder and saw that all remnants of a gothic, hipper Cait were gone. In its place, clad in sneakers and a sweatshirt, was the youthful, struggling teen I knew only too well.

"Come on, Cait. We've only a couple of hours of afternoon light left."

She was already lagging. "My stomach hurts."

How? I had let her fill up on a burger and milkshake at McDonald's before we left so she wouldn't complain about hunger and fatigue.

"Just keep moving. We'll take it slow." No way are you quitting on me.

Normally, I loved the idea of a Sunday hike. But this was different, and the nervous pit in my stomach, whenever it came to Cait and school, continued to grow, even on a beautiful, late summer afternoon like this one.

We had spent the earlier part of the day navigating Google—Cait's new guardian angel. Google Map directions to the mountain led us one exit south, off the interstate, from her school. It was going to be a piece of cake to find, but I forgot that all side roads in Vermont eventually reverted to dirt. My directions had us veering off one way, while road signs suggested another. Fortunately, Sunday-afternoon dog walkers came to our rescue, each one modifying the directions enough to keep us climbing with a false sense that we were getting closer to our destination.

"This is crazy," I muttered. We passed several places that vaguely looked like a trailhead, but still no signs.

When we reached a T in the road, I'd had enough. "Right turn or left?"

She shrugged, "How would I know?"

"Had you gone on the damn field trip in the first place you would!"

Silence.

I turned right. As I kept driving, I thought I heard what sounded like a desperate voice repeating the same mantra, "I can't believe I'm doing this," until I recognized it as my own.

"Okay, if we don't find it after the next bend, I'm turning around." Great. Just what I need—to drive to the ends of the Earth, get lost, and still never get to the damn trailhead.

The next bend came, but I kept going. Something deep down in me wouldn't give up. Our perseverance paid off as we turned the corner and were rewarded with cars announcing the trail entrance. We made it with a couple of hours of daylight to spare.

The path was well traveled. We kept passing hikers moving down the mountain, headed back to their cars. It didn't matter. I knew the lab wouldn't be easy to complete without doing the climb. Every time I looked her way, her face was unreadable. I couldn't gage her investment.

I began to wonder about what other detour signs would spring up that semester. I still couldn't be certain of what Cait would accomplish once back on campus. Her attention could easily drift into other things, causing her to lose all track of time. I imagined the conversation inside her head, "Now what was I supposed to be doing?" Other times, I think she knew the drill and simply avoided it, like the hike. It was as though there were two of her, the Cait who wanted to be mature and successful and the one who escaped into her cyber-connected world where hours evaporated. If I'd beg the question, "Why not put college on hold for a while or attend the community college, a class at a time?" she'd become adamant, "I can do this," she'd assert.

That's how she'd suck me back in. I wanted to believe in her. I knew how much campus life meant. Even if she existed only on the fringe, she was part of something she'd never experienced before. I always found myself continuing to root for the Cait who wanted to make this work.

As we continued along the trail, I made her stop to take mental notes of her surroundings: species of trees, glacial evidence, dominant plants. I began thinking about how I'd teach the course myself.

Amazingly, my anxiety began to subside, much like the ache in Cait's stomach. Her energy returned and I'd find her stopping to collect seeds for another class project. She started rattling off the names of the trees and shrubs. That's my Cait.

As we got closer to the top, our efforts paid off. I gave myself a moment to breathe. We had a 180-degree, panoramic picture of the Connecticut Valley, which spread out like a quilted blanket below. Autumn had touched down and painted some of the trees crimson. I could sense Cait felt it, too. When we finally reached the very top, a wide circle of raised, flat stones, our very own Stonehenge, greeted us. To celebrate her success, Cait danced around them, like a sprite, tracing their path.

We weren't alone. An older gentleman was posed on one of the rocks, sitting stock still with his feet stretched out in front of him and his eyes closed, facing the last rays of the day. Next to him, carefully placed, were his pack and walking stick. I wondered what path he'd traveled and how far he had walked. He blended in so perfectly, we almost didn't see him at first. Though his slight frame and staff hinted at his age, his face was smooth and tanned. His eyes remained closed the whole time we were there. I envied his serenity and ability to shut out the world around him. Cait could often do the same, while other times she was a whirligig.

I turned and suggested she take some shots with her phone camera, proof she'd been there. This time, as we walked back down the trail, she led the way. My nervous pit had vanished. The day morphed back into the beautiful late summer day it was—perfect for a mother and daughter jaunt up Black Mountain.

29

SAVING CAIT

After her Black Mountain fiasco, Cait understood the importance of not missing another field trip. She was beginning to find her rhythm. A bigger, more important assignment was coming up, climbing Mount Monadnock, a three-thousand-plus-footer. It would take all day, and would require an excused absence from other classes. Her teacher prepped them on clothing and gear, water and food, as October could be extremely windy and cold. They'd be exploring the alpine flora and identifying lichen along the way. Cait was pumped. The weekend before the hike she had come home and pulled together all the essentials. She even asked me to buy extra snacks to share.

When I dropped her off that Sunday, before Monday's trip, we practiced the drill. "Remember, set your alarm. Set both your phone and clock alarms. Don't take any chances."

"I know. I know."

I watched her slowly walk toward her dorm, weighted down with the weekend's extras. I couldn't stop myself from calling out, "You can even pack your stuff tonight so it will be ready."

She looked back and nodded.

The following morning as I drove to work I had an unexpected text from her. She was already up and ready. As soon as I got to school, I called to wish her good luck. "Don't forget to meet them in the parking lot, have a great time. I love you."

"Back at you."

Her excitement and the cloudless sky made me believe that everything was all right. She was headed down the right path this time.

Throughout the morning I found myself looking at the clock and wondering where she might be right then. If they had left campus at nine o'clock, they'd likely be arriving at the trailhead around ten. It was probably a good thirty- to forty-five-minute drive. Is she sitting with anyone on the bus? Striking up a conversation? On the trail will her instructor praise her quick eye and enthusiasm? She could use the brownie points.

Earlier in the term when we met with her advisor, she shared that Cait was often rude and abrupt with her science instructor. While Cait was surprised, I was furious. I knew that Cait was not always aware of her tone and that her comments could be offensive, but I expected her to tow the line. I also recognized that this class came just as her a.m. meds were wearing off. Not a good combination. We had the "talk" and decided to do a little adjusting with the meds. As we left her advisor's office that day I asked, "Cait, what gives? This is a favorite subject for you. Why so snappy with your teacher?"

"I don't know. Abigail is just *too perky*."

"Seriously? Too perky??" Our eyes locked and we suddenly cracked up at what was apparently a major crime in Cait's book of top-ten offensives. Unfortunately, her instructor had her own book of top ten.

Later that morning, as I was calf deep in a nearby rushing stream with my fourth graders searching for elusive crayfish, my cell phone buzzed. When I flipped it open, I had a voice mail. I assumed it was the school secretary. It was far from the voice I was expecting.

"Hi Mom, it's me, Cait." Her voice sounded distant and small. "I messed up big time. I thought the bus was leaving at ten," barely catching her breath she continued, "I went and waited for it at the wrong time. I missed the bus."

Not again.

"I was supposed to get there at nine and now I don't know what to do. I just really need someone to help me right now." In a click she was gone.

The sounds of the stream and children's voices seemed warped and out of sync. I worked my way over to our class assistant. "I just got a call from Cait. It's an emergency. I have to call her right back. Please keep an eye on things." As I fumbled to make the call, all I could think was that I needed someone to help me right now, too.

Cait picked up almost immediately. I couldn't hold back my own flood of words. "I can't believe it. Oh my God, Cait, how did you miss the bus? Didn't you remember the time?"

Obviously she didn't, so why was I asking? The irony of her being ready at the crack of dawn and missing the bus was over the top.

She was crying on the other end. I crumbled, "I'm so sorry, Cait. I know how much you wanted to go on this. Get to your advisor right now and tell her what happened. Hurry. Just go and find her."

I shut the phone and turned to my class. "We have to head back now." I ignored their moans and grumbles. The short walk back up the hill to our classroom felt like the longest of my life. My mind was flooded. If I leave right now, could I get her to the trailhead? Sure like I could get someone who missed their flight up to their plane in mid-air.

I was convinced this most recent screw up couldn't be salvaged. Cait had already been cited for her class attitude, and now a third of the way into the term, she had missed two field trips. This had to place her on "the most likely to fail list."

As the day wore on, I was overcome with my own guilt. After all the endless drilling, I'd never thought to double-check the time with her, even when we spoke that morning. I confided to my assistant more than once that day, "If only I had called at 8:30 and asked her if she was heading for the parking lot. God, if I'd done that, she'd be on that hike right now."

But her reason for screwing up the departure time became clearer to me as the day wore on. Mondays she had communications class at ten. That's what she had had to forfeit for the hike. Her brain was fixed on Mondays at ten. What took weeks to permanently etch in her mind was now set. She was on automatic pilot. The schedule she had painstakingly learned, brought her crashing down in the end.

Miraculously, Cait did reach her advisor in her office. It was clear this wasn't the case of a missed alarm, or a feeble excuse for not participating. Her advisor connected with her instructor the next day and informed Cait that Abigail wanted to meet with her—a hopeful sign. Abigail gave Cait two choices: Make up the field lab by getting the information from a classmate, or take the hike.

So though I would find myself on a different mountain and trail this time, the mission remained the same—saving Cait.

30

MOUNTAIN THAT STANDS ALONE

The next Sunday at ten, Cait and I were in the parking lot of the Dublin Trail. "Okay, it's 2.2 miles to the summit. Hopefully, no more than a couple of hours at best."

The day before, the two of us had labored over lichen cards making for easier identification and hopefully a seamless trip. As we started up the mountain, people were already passing us on their way down, a good sign. This will be even quicker than I thought. Or so difficult they're already bailing! No way was I sharing my worry.

"This isn't so bad, Cait. We even have a sunny day." I cheerfully yelled back to her.

No comment.

She held onto the straps of her backpack, head down, sidestepping rocks. She was saving her breath.

We hadn't gone even a couple of feet when I heard her stop behind me. "Wait, there's a lichen on this tree. I need to write it down." She whipped out her stack of lichen cards. As I stepped towards her, I slipped and quickly caught a nearby branch to steady myself. The trail was slick and muddy from a recent rainstorm and I couldn't stop thinking about the miles that stretched ahead of us.

How the hell did I end up here? I am either the world's best mom or its biggest idiot.

Our morning energy kept us pumped. Cait's cheeks were already rosy and her eyes alert, and bright. She had us stopping frequently in front of rock outcroppings and tree trunks so she could log her findings. As much as I wanted to quicken our pace, I was glad to see her taking the hike seriously. I wished she had been able to share it with her classmates instead of me.

The climb was steady and slow, and Cait was still behind me, moving. Sometimes when she stopped to look at something, she wouldn't call ahead, so I'd have to backtrack only to discover her mesmerized. "Look at this!"

As the trail narrowed and got steeper, we clung to tree branches and pulled ourselves along in search of secure footholds among the slippery rocks. As we shifted from hardwood to dense hemlock forest, I kept checking the time. "Cait, we've still got a stretch to go. We're not even above tree line. You need to pick it up."

"Okay, okay," she grumbled back.

As though the mountain read my mind, scenic vistas began to emerge making our slow efforts finally pay off. But along with the dramatic views of the valley below came the granite boulders, Monadnock's trademark. We became human mountain goats as we crawled steadily up and over the rocks.

Focused solely on my footing, I was suddenly jolted by a piercing cry from behind. Cait was down, and clinging to her ankle with huge crocodiles tears. Oh crap.

In an instant other hikers magically appeared and made their way over to her voicing their concerns.

"Are you okay?"

"Can you move your ankle?"

"Keep it straight."

"Don't take your shoe off, it will swell and you won't be able to get back down the mountain."

I was grateful, but overwhelmed by their advice. I imagined waiting for the trail's rescue brigade, towing an orange stretcher and medic bag, or a helicopter trying to land on a nonexistent flat boulder, but most of all, I imagined Cait not completing the damn lab. I was quickly losing my status of super mom. I found my voice, "Cait, you'll be okay. Give your ankle a minute to rest."

I turned to our Samaritans. "Thanks you so much. I'm *sure* she'll be fine." They scattered as quickly as they had gathered.

I sat down along side her. The tears had stopped and were replaced with whimpers.

"Cait, we can stop here or try to make it the rest of the way. It's not that much further. Why don't you see if you can put some pressure on it?"

She looked at me as though I had taken leave of my senses.

"Come on, I'll help you."

I got up and pulled her dead weight to an upright position. "Let's try going just a little further." I found myself pleading, "Come on. We came all this way."

"It hurts," she whined. With more coaxing, she hobbled a little ahead, but not without throwing the grumpiest scowl she could muster my way. I had undoubtedly just entered her "perky" offense zone.

I think she surprised us both by continuing, albeit slowly, over the remaining rocks. Not long after we reached the top, we were greeted by intense winds. It would take us another fifteen minutes to climb to the summit, but we made it. We passed on climbing the rest of the way to the peak, and instead hunkered down behind a large boulder and pulled out our lunch. It was too cold for anything more than a few bites of sandwich. When I tried to speak, my words were lost in the gusts of cold air. We ended up sitting silently, side-by-side, inviting some of our energy to return.

After lunch we reversed direction. As we started down the path we'd just come up, we sighted a cluster of delicate white alpine flowers tucked just off the trail. I marveled at their tenacity, along with our own. If flowers could still blossom under the cruelest conditions, so could my daughter.

It was slow going. I gave up looking at my watch. We were each lost in our own thoughts. At one point I chuckled to find Cait sliding down the rocks on her bottom. A little further down I heard her cry out. Now what?

But when I checked, I found her turned around, exposing a huge, gaping tear in her pants.

"Geez, Cait." We suddenly broke down laughing, one of those deep belly laughs, while we voiced how grateful we were to perky Abigail for her advice on layering.

We made it back to the car bone tired. I felt dirty and chilled and wanted a hot shower more than anything. But we weren't done. Cait needed to complete the lab and report her observations. I didn't dare leave it to chance.

Before I dropped her off, we stopped at a local burger joint where she could be buoyed with another hamburger and shake. Our feet stuck to the gummy floor as we searched for a clean table to spread out books and laptop. When we felt satisfied that the work was complete, we piled back into the car and I dropped Cait off.

That night, after two aspirin, I crawled under the covers and wondered about the effects the hike would have on my weary bones the next day, yet I was content that Cait had gotten over one more hurdle. Earlier in the week I had come across the Abenaki meaning for Monadnock—"Mountain That Stands Alone" —a fitting name for Cait's journey, except for the times when I was there to travel with her.

31

UNDERSTANDING AND SPEAKING DOG

I stopped the car next to our newspaper box on our way out of the driveway. "Cait, can you get the paper?"

"Sure." She stuck her arm out the window but it didn't reach the box. She quickly undid her seatbelt and half hung out of the car, finally grabbing it. While still horizontal, she started to unroll the paper to read the headlines.

"Cait!"

"Okay, okay." She slithered back in, just clearing her head through the car's window frame. Of course, it would have been a lot easier to just get out of the car, but not for Cait. It always made me crazy, but I knew I'd miss the silly routine and all her antics. As soon as she was buckled, she rifled through the paper looking for the funnies.

I had grown used to Cait riding next to me, telling me when it was okay to change lanes, or whether I had parked too close to the curb. She was my wingman, much like I'd been hers all these years. During summer vacations we'd done some serious traveling together. Once, while visiting Courtney in Boulder, Colorado, we decided to drive across the state of Wyoming to visit Yellowstone and the Tetons. It was a wild road trip. We covered a lot of desolate miles to reach our destination.

Occasionally, Cait would lift her eyes from her Game Boy long enough to take in the next stretch of road. "Look at that sign. Can you believe it? Moneta, population ten!"

"God, where would we stop for gas?"

"Don't worry, your tank is full. I've been watching it." It was her attempt to calm my nerves.

"Thanks, Cait." It was nice to switch roles for a change.

She never complained, even when trapped in the car for hours, despite my habit of stopping to take yet another picture every few miles. "Again? You promised ice cream soon. You don't want us to die of starvation, do you?" And then she'd laugh and go back to her book. My mother had it right. She was a comfort to me. Cait was fun to be around.

Over the years, we had other adventures. When I turned fifty, she was the only family member willing to help me fulfill my dream of riding a train across country to the Pacific. We danced together in the waves when we got there. For two summers, while she was in high school we traveled to the Pacific Northwest, where we watched orcas and explored glaciers. The beauty of the natural world was never lost on her. She could be on the deck of a boat for hours, refusing to go inside afraid there would be some mammal or bird she'd miss. When I look back, I am glad it was Cait riding shotgun. We were a good team, and God knows we'd been through a lot of difficult times together. Having the chance to share those special moments helped me accept the others, the ones that tested my patience, my strength, my ability to problem solve. I can still see myself sitting across the table from Dr. Cooper when Cait was barely four. He told me that her wild spirit could have won her the West. He was right. Cait loved uncharted ground and there was still a lot left to conquer. With the car packed, we were heading into new territory again, but only as far west as Burlington, Vermont, this time, where twenty-three years earlier Cait had first entered our lives, beginning our story, on a sunny and beautiful day like this one.

"So this is it, Cait. Excited?"

She was plugged into her iPod, humming, but I knew, if she chose to, she could still hear me. She did. "Yes, yes, yes!"

"Me, too." I smiled, stretching the truth. I was a mix of emotions, but anxious and sad seemed to be trumping the others.

Weeks earlier she'd decided to have her hair highlighted, and after a summer of activity, her skin, usually pale, had gained a tan glow. The new look inched her a little closer to her actual age.

It made me a little more confident in what we were about to do. I had rallied around this day for as long as I knew my daughter. But this was different from launching her off to college. I was sending her off to a new life, and other than holidays and vacations, I doubted she'd be back.

Earlier that spring Cait had graduated college, getting her associates degree. Like most things in Cait's life, participation had to be at her speed. After that first year, she never carried a full course load, eventually making it to the end, with plenty of help. A small family contingent was there to share her moment.

"Cait!" Courtney called out to her as she and the other grads gathered in front of the building for pictures before lining up.

She waved back, ecstatic. She was positioned up front and as cameras clicked, I remembered back to the elementary school class shot and how she seemed to fit right in with her peers. This was no different. You couldn't tell that she came home almost every weekend to lay out her books as we scrutinized each assignment or that on the ride back on Sunday afternoons I'd drill her on what she needed to do that week. I was convinced I had single-handedly chipped away at the independence I craved for her, yet it was the only way I knew to get her through.

Courtney and I sat up front next to my dad and Mike, and watched as the graduates filed in and took their places on stage next to the podium. Cait was right in the first row, poised and ready for the large audience facing her, until she whipped out a rubber stress ball letting it fly in our direction. It barely missed the head of an elderly white-haired woman in the seat next to mine. "Cait!" I cried out, as she laughed. But once the crowd quieted down, so did our graduate. And for the next couple of hours she hung in, listening to countless speeches and eventually walking up to receive her diploma. It was another Cait milestone. But what next?

As we passed by the late summer black-eyed Susans growing wild on the edge of the highway, Cait settled back into her music silently signaling, "No more questions."

We were headed to a program that had been designed to support young adults with developmental disabilities, like Asperger's. Cait would be living in a house with other students, just blocks away from the University of Vermont campus, taking classes specifically designed for developing communication and life skills. The program encouraged students to take classes at a local college, but with a light load and ever-present support for both living and studying.

The day Cait received the call telling us she was accepted, I felt like we won the lottery. It was state funded. I saved the message on my machine and played it back all week. I had wanted independence for Cait as long as I could remember, and now someone else, besides me, was stepping in to help her achieve it.

Our car was less packed this time as the new program provided lots of essentials. But would they provide everything she'd need? No matter where Cait landed there was always a built-in learning curve for anyone involved with my daughter: different routines, periods of adjustment, new crises. As we continued the drive, Cait's eyes were closed and she was humming. How did those years of rocking her in the early dawn hours disappear so quickly? And how did we get through the intervening years, to this place, to this moment of cutting the umbilical tether?

When we arrived at the Burlington house, it was filled with young people. The program was based around mentorship. What better way to learn social cues than by modeling them. Though some staff members were older, most were recent UVM grads. This time, as Cait and I emptied her belongings out of the car, we had help at every turn. As she settled in, staff stopped by to see what they could do: hang a picture, help unpack, move furniture, anything to make it more comfortable. It was an older house with a lot of character and a leather couch that faced a flat-screen TV in the living room. I was jealous. The kitchen was completely equipped and there was even a washer and dryer. No more traveling to the Laundromat with Cait on Saturday mornings.

Once she was unpacked, she was eager for me to take off. I understood. I didn't feel the need to call every day making sure she was up for class or that she passed her English paper in. Someone else would do that, and eventually, Cait would fend for herself. I was leaving her in good hands. She seemed ready to make some serious inroads toward self-reliance. As I drove off, a huge weight on my shoulders lifted.

It was October and Cait and I strolled along the path that bordered Lake Champlain taking in the Adirondack peaks in the distance. I had brought our family dog, Maggie. Cait hadn't been home since late August. Her stepdad and I had visited her a month earlier, bringing bikes to ride along the same path. Now it was just Maggie and me checking in on her. She looked great. "How are things going? Your classes?"

"Really good."

"Tell me about them."

"I love the dog class. The teacher brings in different breeds each week." She was gushing.

Cait had signed up for a continuing education class at UVM entitled, Understanding and Speaking Dog. It was as if it had been designed just for her. Since she had been old enough to crawl, she'd had a passion for four-legged creatures. The only glitch was the timing. It was offered on Wednesday evenings and was three-and-a-half-hours long. Happily, though, a staff member met her when it was over so she wouldn't have to walk home alone in the dark.

"Do you eat before you go to class?"

"Yeah, but sometimes I bring a sandwich with me."

We continued our walk in silence for a little.

Suddenly Cait shared, "I was surprised last week in class."

"Really?"

"We had a quiz."

"How'd you do?"

"I think okay."

The light bulb had now officially been lit and Cait had turned the switch.

The following morning I shot the project manager an email. "Cait shared she was surprised by a recent quiz." I couldn't help myself. "I'm assuming someone's checking in with her." I figured at this point Cait was motivated enough to take some responsibility for her assignments, but at the same time, I recognized she needed support in all aspects of her new environment, including her classes.

When Cait entered the program I had decided I wasn't going to micromanage from two hours away. They seemed to have every necessary fail-safe in place. I explained to the staff the most important thing they'd need to know about Cait: Don't believe her. It's not that she's a liar, it's just that she prefers to work undercover. To Cait, everything is fine, "really." I learned the right response years ago. "Show me."

When something gets overwhelming, Cait doesn't admit to it or ask for help. It will make its appearance in other ways: more time online, sleeping late, picking at her skin, grumpiness, teary outbursts over a pet that died five years ago. The fact that she dropped me a clue that day was extraordinary.

The project manager assured me she'd look into it.

A day later I got a phone call from Cait. "Mom, I need your charge number to order some books."

"Books? What for?"

"For one of my classes. You know, the dog one."

It was October and the class had started at the end of August.

"Cait, is someone there I can speak to?"

It was worse than I had imagined. She was already weeks in and hadn't even purchased one book. Four were required. It turned out the quiz she was referring to happened each week and was based on the readings. The class was lecture-based and the lectures formed the basis for periodic exams. Unfortunately, the university's Disability Services hadn't included a notetaker in her accommodations. Cait had successfully turned in a paper on her favorite dog breed, the springer, but it wasn't enough for her to pass.

Finally, a staff member accompanied her to class to assess the damage. She reported back that the class was busy, very busy. Several dogs were brought in weekly, providing a good bit of distraction, while lots of information was disseminated. She concluded that after the first two hours, Cait was fried.

Who could I blame? From August until October I was free as a bird. The times I had wanted to ask and dig a little, I had held back. It was someone else's turn. From their end, Cait had a handle on all her other classes, which were offered through their program (straight As, even in her personal finance class), though I later learned that she had spent all her book money on a life-size stuffed reptile, clothing from Second Time Around, junk food, and an exotic gold cane for Halloween. It's safe to say her mother would have given her a big, fat F in personal finance. I suppose everyone figured her university class was going equally well. They listened and never looked—a big mistake. I remembered my own learning curve back at Cait's college, but at least she'd had a scholarship then. This mistake ended up costing me $1,600—the cost of a university course. Cait did finish out the class, but only through a team effort: the university's ACCESS department, her project manager and I were able to turn it from a three-credit course to an audit as most of the deadlines had passed. My biggest worry was that Cait would end up failing at what she was passionate about. Although she gleaned a lot about dog behavior from her work with Elsa and Echo, the therapy dog, as well as from her addiction to *Animal Planet*, there was still a lot more to learn, and it saddened me that she was missing out.

The team plugged her into volunteering at a local shelter for rescue dogs and she scored an internship at the nearby aquatic science center the following fall. My fingers were now permanently frozen in a crossed position. I hoped she could keep the momentum going.

Although things seemed to be heading in the right direction, "hiccups" were always a part of Cait's life. There was no rule book, no map. Sometimes, it was a little like crossing the state of Wyoming, where sparsely placed road signs signaled, "Next exit 100 miles." Do I have enough fuel to make it? Do I believe the girl who's next to me telling me not to worry? Maybe someday they'll have a course to prepare you. It would have to be titled, Understanding and Speaking Cait. But as far as I know, I don't think it's in the offing anytime soon. They're still working on Asperger's 101.

EPILOGUE

THE FLEDGLING

Cait, now twenty-four, continues to live in Burlington, taking classes in her program and pursuing work experiences. I often worry about her future and where it will all lead. She still seems so young and innocent that I can't imagine her out on her own. But don't all parents feel that way?

I remember back to the spring that she turned sixteen, when our house became home to a pair of phoebes. Though we'd been living there for close to two decades, they seemed to have just discover us. The nest magically appeared one day, wedged on top of an outdoor thermometer, beyond the doorway leading from our kitchen to a small patio and flower garden. Their refuge, perfectly packed with mud and grass, held four nestlings that year.

I was honored they chose us and instructed everyone to avoid the doorway. I abandoned gardening so as not to disturb their now busy family life. Yet as suddenly as they arrived, they were gone. Were we away the day their babies were launched? Could it be that quick or that easy?

At summer's end, I convinced my family the nest should stay put. On those winter days when cold air blasted out of the north, our thermometer, encased with summer mud and straw, kept us all guessing exactly how cold it was. My family thought I was crazy for protecting a vacant nest, but I was possessed with this unreasonable logic that if they returned and their home was gone, they'd choose another place to live.

One afternoon in late May I arrived home from work to discover their old nest lying on the bench below. My first thought was wind, but after surviving the winter's nor'easters I knew better. I found Cait reading in her room, "What happened to the nest?" I was unreasonably annoyed.

She hesitated for one second too long. "I don't know," then shrugged and looked back at her story.

I turned to leave. "I know you moved it, Cait."

Later that evening, as I was preparing dinner, she came quietly into the kitchen and sat down at the table. "I thought I'd move it to a place where they'd be more likely to find it."

"Cait, they'll never build on the bench. They'd be too vulnerable there." So after a year of safekeeping, I was now certain they wouldn't come back, and I knew that Cait felt my disappointment, too. She enjoyed their presence more than any of us.

Several days later, we came downstairs one morning and to our amazement found a pair of phoebes rebuilding in the exact same spot. Soft, downy heads again emerged, but this year would be different.

The start of that summer was wet and cold, and one rainy day we discovered a fledgling with its soft new feathers on the patio below. Pushed out too soon? The local bird sanctuary advised us to return it to the nest. They explained phoebes wouldn't abandon their young even if humans intervened.

It was no easy task. Teetering below the nest on a small stepladder, I gingerly reached above my head and tried placing the baby bird back as Cait steadied me from below

"Oh, no!" Cait screeched as several more fledglings bounded out onto the patio. It seemed the nest had shrunk or the others had grown too big and were now eager to make their own escape. We scrambled trying to place them back, one at a time, but as soon as we thought they were all safely tucked in, one by one they'd bounce out again. And then the rains came, in torrents. I tried placing them in a shoebox on the bench under the porch's overhang, but even that couldn't contain them.

We understood fair or not, nature runs its own course. We caught sight of the parents nearby but their role became unclear. One parent stayed near the bench never leaving. I listened to the rain's steady rhythm and watched the droplets slide down the summer foliage leaving small puddles on the stones. For a couple of miserable days we kept track of them. In the end, we found two dead fledglings near the patio. We buried them in the same garden where they might have thrived.

I remained haunted by their fate and my part in it. Should I have left the one that first fell out alone? Had these babies fledged too soon, making failure to thrive almost certain? Is there a right time for fledglings to leave the nest, one that guarantees survival, or is survival merely luck? I suppose phoebes have a rhythm that they instinctively understand—how long to feed, when to coax, when it's safe to leave. And perhaps they accept the unexpected. The phoebes reminded me of my own daughter and of that simple lesson: not everything can be controlled, no matter a parent's best effort.

So many times, I had believed Cait was ready to move ahead when she wasn't. Just when I thought we had reached the finish line, something would come along and shift it.

"You still have several more miles to go, Cait."

"But I'm out of breath" she would say—and I would reply, "It doesn't matter."

But it did.

I thought I had found the perfect program for her in Burlington to foster her independence and finally launch her out into the world, but once out of the nest, she still floundered.

Her sister, Courtney, lives in Maine now. She works at a university not far from the coast, and chooses to live off the mainland on a small island. She tells us she doesn't mind the ferry ride each day. It gives her a chance to reflect. Cait and I have visited Courtney's island home several times. Some of its isolated beaches have the most amazing sea glass that dapples the sand in blues and greens. I can't help but think it's the wrong daughter living there; after all, isn't it Courtney who flourishes around people? She has groups of friends in every city she's ever visited. Cait is the one who's supposed to run barefoot and free. Wouldn't the island offer her an easier path? I imagine Cait driving around in a golf cart, much like the ones on Cuttyhunk, pet sitting the dogs of wealthy summer guests or making things to sell from her beach treasures. Instead, she's the one in a small city; still trying to manage the requirements for another college class, speculating whether to spend all her money on a velvet cape that catches her eye, or working hard to hold up her end of the conversation when she's looking for a job. On our last visit to Courtney's, I watched several gulls safely land on the shoreline's jagged rocks and remembered our lost phoebes.

At the end of the summer, all those years back, we took down the second phoebe nest. Soon after, the house was painted. The thermometer came off and wasn't replaced. I never admitted to anyone the depth of my sadness—a sadness that left me wondering about my own daughter's fate and her numerous attempts to fledge. I know now that the readiness of an Apserger's child is not guaranteed and parents operate in a void trying to gauge what they might expect. No matter how reasonable we think the expectation is, it isn't. Failures at flight far outnumber the successes. We find ourselves hopeful, but secretly recognize that things may not go right.

Still, the phoebes taught me something profound. The fledglings that bounded out of the nest that day were daring, resilient little birds. Not all the baby birds perished. Some flew off. They survived.

Cait has never complained about where she's landed or that she's discouraged or lonely or sad. She has never stopped plugging along, happily rounding the next corner, and understanding more than any of us that this is her journey. Maybe that's where the lesson lies. Like the birds in our garden, she'll be home in the springtime, open to trying again. And like the mother phoebe, I need to be patient and ready to embrace my daughter's next season.

Made in the USA
Charleston, SC
24 July 2014